INFERTILITY IN A
CROWDED COUNTRY

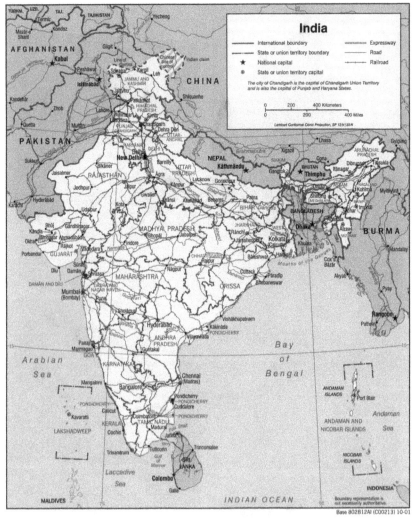

Figure a.1. Map of India, 2001. Library of Congress, Geography and Map Division.

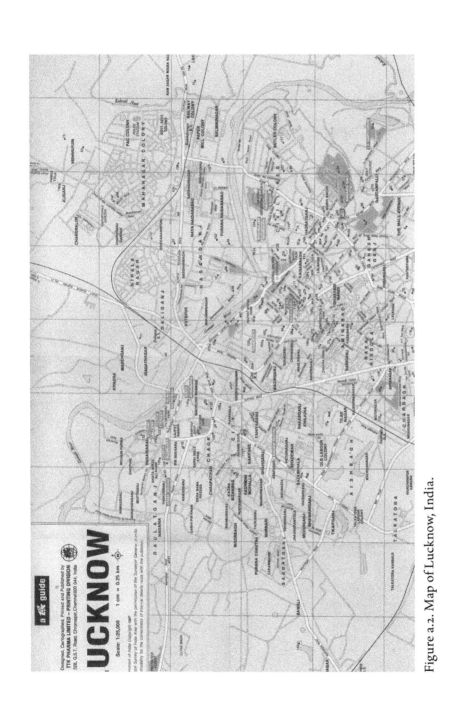

Figure a.2. Map of Lucknow, India.

INFERTILITY IN A
CROWDED COUNTRY

Hiding Reproduction in India

—⁓—

Holly Donahue Singh

INDIANA UNIVERSITY PRESS

This book is a publication of

Indiana University Press
Office of Scholarly Publishing
Herman B Wells Library 350
1320 East 10th Street
Bloomington, Indiana 47405 USA

iupress.org

Manufactured in the United States of America

First printing 2022

Cataloging information is available from the Library of Congress.

ISBN 978-0-253-06386-1 (hardback)
ISBN 978-0-253-06387-8 (paperback)
ISBN 978-0-253-06388-5 (ebook)

For Anushka and those growing with her around the world, in honor of those who have traveled on.

CONTENTS

ACKNOWLEDGMENTS

BOOKS IN THE SOCIAL SCIENCES inevitably gather debts as they come into being. This book is certainly no exception. More than two decades have passed since I traveled from the United States to India on my very first plane ride, at the beginning of a trip that, unbeknownst to me, would set in motion a career. On its way to the present avatar, this project has taken many forms. As a writer, a scholar, and a researcher, I have been fortunate to have the blessing of presenting and discussing my work with many interlocutors, mentors, teachers, fellows, and friends over years and across thousands of miles of travels. They include the staff who managed the spaces and finances that have enabled my work, the caregivers who freed me for scholarship, and all who have helped me along the travels, moves, many career stages, and innumerable cups of chai. These contributions are essential to academic work, yet often remain invisible. As a scholar from a working-class and sometimes poor family, I would be remiss not to recognize their support.

First and foremost, my thanks and infinite gratitude go to the people in India who have shared their lives and their stories with me, creating the possibility of this book and the foundations for my continuing efforts as a scholar and as a human being. Inevitably, despite my best efforts and in order to protect the confidentiality of my interlocutors and the people they put me in contact with in India who shared some of their most closely held stories, many will miss mention by name here. They may well recognize themselves in the text: social activists, medical professionals, teachers, students, people experiencing infertility, family members. For not recognizing them by name, I beg their forgiveness, their understanding, and their patience. Without them, this work and my career as a scholar could not be. Despite their best efforts, the responsibility for the remaining deficiencies in my analysis remains with me. I offer the text that follows as part of a journey toward better clarity in understanding the complexities of fertility and family on this small orb we all share, however small or large our physical or social space within it may be.

I would like to thank everyone who has commented on and responded to my work during the course of conferences and guest talks too numerous to list here, and which would surely be incomplete. Among them, Marcia Inhorn and the other organizers of and participants in Reproductive Disruptions: Childlessness, Adoption, and Other Reproductive Complexities at the University of Michigan in 2005 and Anindita Majumdar and the team that hosted Reframing the Biological Clock: Exploring Ageing and Reproduction in Contemporary Ethnographies in 2018 at the Indian Institute of Technology, Hyderabad, India, stand out as organizers of bookending events for this project's inspiration to begin and to finish. Contributors to the Annual Conference on South Asia, Feminist Pre-Conference, and the American Institute of Indian Studies' dissertation-to-book workshop; the American Anthropological Association and Society for Applied Anthropology; and the Population Association of America (PAA) annual meetings have also generously offered feedback. I am grateful to the anonymous reviewers who dedicated their time to providing thorough and thoughtful feedback for improving the manuscript and to the wonderful editorial and other staff at

Indiana University Press for seeing this book through completion and into the world, with special thanks to my kind and generous editor Jennika Baines, assistant editor Sophia Hebert, and director Gary Dunham.

Since 2017, I have been working as a faculty member at the University of South Florida's Judy Genshaft Honors College amid a buzzing community of undergraduate students, faculty, and staff who keep me engaged with their enthusiasm, questions, and curiosity about my work. Students Yesha Shukla and Sarah Lendavay both commented on the manuscript and helped in its preparation. The Department of Anthropology has also welcomed me into their intellectual community, as I encourage Honors students to explore what anthropology and related social science and humanistic endeavors have to offer. They are all wonderful in their own ways and deserving of recognition, most especially another Honors faculty member who started the journey with me, Ulluminair Salim, and her daughter, Nadira. Before Tampa, I found a home for one charmed year as an Andrew W. Mellon Postdoctoral Fellow in Anthropology at Bowdoin College in Brunswick, Maine. Engaging with my colleagues there proved crucial for many reasons, and special thanks are due to Nancy Riley, Sara Dickey, Krista Van Vleet, Divya Gupta, Vyjayanthi Ratnam Selinger, Tricia Welsch, Rachel Sturman, student assistant Ari Mehrberg, and Gary Lawless and Beth Leonard, among many other friends we made on campus and off during that brief, intense year.

This book benefited greatly from the intellectual, financial, and institutional support of the Population Studies Center (PSC) at the Institute for Social Research, University of Michigan. A postdoctoral training fellowship funded by the National Institute for Child Health and Human Development (training grant T32 HD007339 and center grant R24 HD041028) under the NICHD-Kirschstein Postdoctoral Training program afforded me precious nonteaching time to focus on the publication of my work, while expanding and deepening my interdisciplinary connections with other scholars of family, health, and social issues. I thank my mentor, Tom Fricke, and other members of the Institute for Social Research at Michigan for bringing me into their community, and for offering me space, time, and resources to write and to continue my research program. Special thanks go to the other postdoctoral scholars at the PSC and in the Department of Anthropology, especially Apoorva Jadhav, Emily Smith-Greenaway, Yasmin Moll, and Sarah Besky. My time in Ann Arbor was also enriched by working with two enthusiastic undergraduates eager to learn about social science research in India: Nayna Rath and Prachi Bharadwaj.

Colleagues at the University of Notre Dame encouraged me to prioritize my writing and research agenda, despite my position as visiting teaching faculty. The Friday afternoon writing club, under the leadership of Susan Sheridan, served as a regular reminder to make time for my own scholarship amid the constant press of responsibilities to students and to the never-ending rounds of job applications and interviews. Mentors and colleagues at Notre Dame gave generously of their time to think with me about presenting myself and my work. Susan Blum, Agustín Fuentes, and Ian Kujit helped me navigate the university and job market. James McKenna and Carolyn Nordstrom offered their long-term perspectives on managing career, scholarship, and students while keeping self and family going. Meredith Chesson, Gabriel Torres, Jada Benn Torres, and Christopher Ball provided support and encouragement for knowing there would never be a balance of family and work responsibilities, but to keep going anyway. Donna Glowacki lent her ear and helped keep me grounded through a long period of uncertainty. Vania Smith-Oka and Rahul Oka welcomed us to South Bend and offered their advice and companionship. Their daughter, Kalpana, along with other children of the department, folded Anushka into their mix, and other members of the department graciously accepted their play as part of the ambiance of the place. My closest office neighbor, Cynthia Mahmood, shared her writing and her journeys, and invited me to do the same. Without the support of these colleagues, I might have given up on academic anthropology. I thank them for being there and for tolerating my moaning about early-morning classes and the "polar vortex." Jonathan Marks and Agustín Fuentes brought humor and broad views that helped me begin to consider the idea of "integrative anthropology" as it is taking shape. Two undergraduate students, Diana Gutierrez and Mary Schmidt, did valuable work to support my research and my engagement with national organizations. During my time at Notre Dame, Daniel Jordan Smith from Brown University and Jennifer Johnson-Hanks from the University of California, Berkeley, found me and my work and invited me to join a new initiative designed to widen the engagement of anthropologists with interdisciplinary population studies. With their support, and funding from the PAA, Brown, and U-C Berkeley, I attended the PAA meetings and visited Brown's Population Studies and Training Center and Watson Institute for International Studies to begin to explore intersections of my work with population studies and demography, which I deepened at Michigan and through the continuing encouragement of Jan Brunson. Other intrepid and persistent writers have also encouraged me over the years: thank you, Sarah Pinto, Emma Varley, Anindita Majumdar, Siri Suh, Heide Castañeda, Patricia Jeffery, Priya Pramod Satalkar, Deepak and Anushka Singh, the Writing Wizards at the University of Michigan, and faculty writing groups at Bowdoin College and the University of South Florida.

The work represented in this book had its most immediate beginnings in my doctoral work at the University of Virginia (UVA). Coursework in the Anthropology Department and department life in all its richness of long conversations at lectures, during seminar breaks, at parties, at protests for the ongoing campaign for living wages for university workers, and at many other sites of our common endeavors have provided endless provocation for me to examine my work anew in conversations that continue beyond the bounds of my degree and make me hesitate to portray any of these connections as completed or in the past. The department and the Graduate School of Arts and Sciences provided financial support for coursework; language study; preliminary research; and, eventually, dissertation writing. I would be remiss not to acknowledge the contributions of most, if not all, of the faculty, graduate students, administrative staff, and many undergraduate students who have been my fellow travelers in anthropology, with our base in Brooks Hall. First, I would like to thank the members of my dissertation committee. R. S. Khare, Susan McKinnon, and Wende Elizabeth Marshall worked with me from the beginning of the dissertation, Mehr Farooqi joined along the way, and Richard Handler kindly volunteered to join near the end. Hanan Sabea drove us to connect anthropological theory since World War II with current events as the United States threatened and then started armed conflict with Iraq during our class, and, later, when many from the department joined undergraduate students in the struggle for fair wages for university employees. Adria LaViolette gently coaxed master's theses and presentations (our both dreaded and loved P&P, or "Paper and Presentation") from my cohort, despite our dire predictions, and always directed us toward the larger significance of our work, which so often escaped us. Peter Metcalf inspired us through preparing grant applications to fund our work in the field, with few complaints about our drama and anxieties. Fred Damon and John Shepherd always asked the questions no one else expected, and Roy Wagner never failed to put them in a larger, often cosmic, perspective. I am indebted to Roy Wagner for the grace and generosity he displayed while I worked as a grader for him through childbirth in lieu of maternity leave, which did not exist for graduate instructors. H. L. Seneviratne gave gentle encouragement not to shy away from integrating perspectives from European traditions into my analysis, while R. S. Khare continually drew me into and drew out of me additional nuance of local categories and South Asian intellectual currents. And Phil McEldowney offered his curiosity, support, and librarian's expertise all along the way.

Members of my small entering cohort of anthropologists became primary collaborators and sounding boards for ideas, among them Amy Nichols-Belo, David Strohl, and Will Schroeder became especially close friends and colleagues, who were never afraid to challenge my ideas. Other graduate students became community—intellectual and otherwise—which often as not centered on care through food. Clare Terni and Sue Ann McCarty introduced me to The People's Kitchen in my first year at UVA, Sherilynn Colby-Bottel and Matt Bottel hosted many memorable parties, and Roberto Armengol coordinated a veritable army of anthropologists to feed my small but growing family during my not-maternity-leave while I wrote my dissertation. Mieka Brand Polanco nurtured my skin and spirit with her olive oil soap and her advice about working and mothering. Claire Snell-Rood became a classificatory younger sister in dissertating who urged me on. We supported one another and, I think, survived the better for it—this was something much more than the "collegiality" touted when I first visited Charlottesville.

I found multiple homes at UVA, with its wealth of programs in interdisciplinary South Asian languages and cultures that, under the direction of members of the Center for South Asian Studies (CSAS; now part of the Asia Institute), brought scholars of South Asia from all over the world to Charlottesville. Because of these resources, and support provided by the university and by the Foreign Language and Area Studies program, I was able to study Hindi and Urdu in Charlottesville, and spend two summers at the American Institute of Indian Studies center for Urdu language in Lucknow, India. Through CSAS, I found a wide community of scholars of South Asia at UVA, working on language, literature, history, and politics. I am thankful for the financial and intellectual support these programs provided me during my formative period of studies and preparatory work. In particular, Griffith Chaussée, Mehr Farooqi, Anand Dwivedi, and Bimla Gour pushed me to deeper engagement with Hindi and Urdu literary traditions, and Robert Hueckstadt, Peter Hook, and Daniel Lefkowitz peppered me with questions and inspired laugher too. All of them worked with me to develop greater confidence in learning and teaching Hindi and Urdu. Richard Barnett kept me connected with Lucknows past and present and reminded me again and again of the importance of both *adab* (good manners) in my conduct, and good headlines in my scholarship. Abdulaziz Sachedina helped me connect my scholarship with wider Islamic and Islamicate worlds of Muslim life and conversations about ethics. The faculty and administrative leaders of CSAS facilitated these interactions by securing funding and keeping the program vital even when funding difficulties arose, especially Daniel Ehnbom, Cindy Benton-Groener, John Nemec, and Richard Cohen. The Program in Studies in Women and Gender at UVA, with the support of Reena Williams, Kath Weston, Geeta Patel, and Laura Mellusi, invited me to teach and thereby allowed me to enrich my work with more explicit connections to gender studies within and beyond anthropology.

Both before and after Virginia, I have benefited from having a home at Kenyon College. As an undergraduate student of the liberal arts, I first encountered subjects as diverse as anthropology, religious studies, and Asian studies. Kenyon professors and students grew me into a person willing to risk going beyond known worlds to explore the world, and then to think, talk, and write about what I found. The mentoring relationships that started during my first year, fresh from the western Pennsylvania farms and fields where I spent my childhood, have continued to the present. I have been blessed with decades of support from Kenyon and from teachers and mentors I also now count as colleagues and friends. Among them, Vernon Schubel and Nurten Kilic-Schubel, Royal Rhodes, David Suggs, Meena Khandelwal, Shuchi Kapila, Joseph Klesner, Clara Roman-Odio, Sam Pack, Kimmarie Murphy, and the late Donald Rogan have played special roles. Wendy Singer, in particular, has guided me tirelessly throughout my scholarly career. Even though I never took a regular course with her at Kenyon, she took me on for an independent study in Hindi and for a summer research project. She also introduced me to Kailash and Abha Jha and their wonderful daughters, Richa and Archita, who became guides, friends, and kin in India and the United States. Don Rogan and his wife, Sally, welcomed me home to Kenyon every time I found my way there, and unfailingly offered kindness and love, while urging me on in my work. I am grateful to the Kenyon village community in its various forms that has encouraged me to follow my curiosity, and then taken supportive interest in the results. Its members have been my most enduring models for teaching and writing.

The webs of social connection anthropologists and others sometimes call networks certainly inform the scholarly work of cultural anthropologists who dare to posit patterns in everyday life, to represent the entwined lives of our interlocutors and ourselves. I am fortunate to have had networks beyond my departments and universities in the United States, especially in Charlottesville, where my intrepid partner in life, Deepak, found his way as a new immigrant from India by making friends among the many South Asians living in central Virginia. Arun and Naina Shah shared many conversations and sandwiches as we all navigated US immigration conventions. We also found many companions from South Asia and from around the world among other families living in the UVA residences at University Gardens and Copeley Hill. Those friendships helped us both a great deal as we dealt with our academic struggles and with the challenges of living between our cultural, social, political, and familial worlds in India and in the United States.

My own geography has been entwined with India since 1998, when I first traveled to Bodh Gaya, the site of the Buddha's enlightenment in Bihar, India, a state that remains close to my heart even as it has moved farther from my research agenda. I started to learn Hindi and meditation as a semester-long student of the Antioch Buddhist Studies program. My first interlocutors and friends in India were and remain from Bihar. A summer research grant from Kenyon and support from my mentors there led me to Lucknow, Uttar Pradesh, the site of the research described in this book, as a Fulbright Scholar from 2000–2001. I have continued to travel there regularly ever since. I have been fortunate to cultivate long-term relationships with many people who have helped to facilitate my research, only some of whom I can name, in the interests of protecting confidentiality. My first introductions to Lucknow came through an Indian Fulbright alumnus (I default here to the more formal Indian system of using honorifics to refer to guides and colleagues), Dr. Roshan Lal Raina, at the Indian Institute of Management (IIM), Lucknow, who introduced me to the city and to his colleagues, and who allowed me to spend time with him and his family at the spacious IIM campus, and to use resources at the IIM Library when I needed a retreat from the city. Under the guidance of Dr. V. D. Pandey, then head of the Department of Medieval and Modern History at Lucknow University, I got the chance of a lifetime to study in Lucknow and, even more significantly, to live at Kailash Hostel, the women's dorm complex for Lucknow University, for over nine months. My profound thanks go to the hostel "warden" at the time, Dr. Nishi Pandey; to the assistant warden, Dr. Nidhi Pandey and her family; and to my fellow hostel "inmates." Among about five hundred students, I was the only foreigner and was glad to be befriended by other young women who were living away from their families. Over the years, I have been glad to find academic support and help in navigating research from others in Lucknow University as well, including Department of Anthropology faculty Drs. Chitralekha

Varma and Indu Sahai, Nadeem Hasnain, and A. P. Singh, and the faculty of the Department of Urdu, especially Dr. Anis Ashfaq Abidi, Dr. M. K. Agarwal of the Dr. Giri Lal Gupta Institute of Public Health, and several doctoral students and alumni of the Urdu program. I met Mr. Ram Advani, the owner of Ram Advani Booksellers and a Lucknow intellectual institution himself, the same day I met my future partner, and he supported us intellectually, professionally, and with his warm personal presence whenever we found ourselves in Lucknow until his passing in 2016. Several prominent social advocates and activists also enabled my work in Lucknow. I honor them here collectively, rather than by name, in the interests of confidentiality. They know their significant contributions, and I know how essential their work is. My work and my career have been enriched by conversations with colleagues and students in India over the years, a debt I recognize and attempt to compensate for by staying in touch and sharing my work in India whenever opportunities to do so arise.

Lucknow has become, for me, a research site and a home, since it is also the hometown of my life partner (*jeevansathi*) and fellow traveler (*humsafar*) Deepak and much of his extended family. We have moved in the United States several times since we formally joined our fortunes in 2002, but we always return to Lucknow. The American Institute of Indian Studies provided me the opportunity to study Urdu language for two summers in Lucknow under the guidance of Dr. Aftab Ahmad, Dr. Jameel Ahmad, Zeba Parveen, Fauzia Farooqui, Rehana Abbasi, and the late Anjum madam. Even before I joined the institute as a student, Dr. A. Y. Mohsin, whom I knew as Akhtar baji, took an interest in me, and I continued to visit her until the summer of 2013, when I appeared on her doorstep only to learn of her passing a short time before. Mrs. Nirmala Sharma, who also passed on in 2013, allowed me to stay both short and long term in her colonial-era bungalow and small guesthouse at Mall Avenue whenever I needed a change or a venue to celebrate—both my wedding and my daughter's first birthday party took place within its boundaries. I learned from Mrs. Sharma, her staff, her friends who joined us for breakfast or dinner from time to time, and fellow guests who tended to be scholars from around the world. At Mrs. Sharma's place, Gauri Shankar, Dinesh, Avdhesh, Mr. Rathore, and Jyoti all provided care, support, and conversation when I needed it. In the grand but crumbling spaces of that Mall Avenue bungalow, I was privileged to meet and dine with people from Lucknow and from around the world who had found their way into Mrs. Sharma's orbit. Sarah Pinto, whom I first met when she was conducting her own doctoral ethnographic project, both challenged me and inspired me.

The American Institute of Indian Studies supported field research for my dissertation project with a junior fellowship from 2006 to 2007. I lived in Lucknow continuously for fourteen months then, with the support of my mentor and "guide" at Lucknow University, the late Dr. Chandralekha Varma. She offered support, connections, a caring ear, and laughter amid the ups and downs of fieldwork. A lifelong resident of Lucknow herself, Dr. Varma produced recommendations that both delighted and confounded me—"Go to the old city, down the road where all the Rastogis [members of a particular caste] live, turn right, find the pharmacy, have someone point out the *peepul* tree, and then ask someone there where to go. You'll find it, no problem." I was skeptical, but she was right. More often than not, I found my way. Over those many months, I found my way into homes, the offices of nongovernmental organizations, medical offices, hospitals, religious sites, schools and colleges, and more and less out-of-the-way places in Lucknow where people invited me to listen and to talk about fertility issues. Many of the people I met along the way, mostly women working as physicians, social workers, and educators, will not see their real names in these pages out of an abundance of caution for their confidentiality and the confidentiality of women they referred me to. Nevertheless, it is their stories and experiences that make this book possible. I give my deepest expression of gratitude to them for allowing me to share some of their most difficult moments with the world, in the interests of better understanding.

At every turn, I have been fortunate to have supporters from my own village near the tiny town of Brockway in rural western Pennsylvania. I grew up surrounded by extended family in a place where many people, whether or not they recognize formal ties of kinship, have known each other's business all too well for generations. All of my parents, siblings, grandparents, and cousins have played important roles in my education and career so far, whether encouraging me; supporting me with words, food, finances, or rides; accepting my choices, even when they seemed unconventional, unwise, or downright foolish from their perspectives; or simply standing aside to allow my journeys to unfold. Even when we have disagreed, as has happened many, many times, I have learned from the experience. My mother, father, stepmother, and maternal grandparents have been my most immediate supporters and sounding boards: Mrs. Wendy Smith, Mr. Rex Donahue, Mrs. Mildred Donahue, Mr. James Grant, and Mrs. Evelyn Grant. My father became ill in August 2015 and fought to recover from a heart attack, stroke, and other complications wrought by a life full of hard times. He died in March of 2016. My teachers, friends, siblings, and other community members know better than I how they have helped me along my way, even as that path took me far away from them again and again.

Since 2002, I have been part of a transnational family. Most of its members have never met one another and can speak together only partially in halting English, so they know each other through photographs and from stories that Deepak and I tell when we visit them. Despite the challenges of always missing someone or the other, dealing with immigration systems, international communication, and travel, my life and my scholarly work have been enriched by this experience. Deepak's parents, Mr. Pavan Kumar Singh and Mrs. Nirmala Singh, his maternal uncles and aunts, Mr. Ganesh Pratap Singh and Mrs. Manorma Singh and Mr. Suresh Pratap Singh and Mrs. Mani Singh, and his siblings Pankaj and, especially, Gunjan, have always kept their hearts and their homes open during our travels. They have given their time, their advice, and their support through our struggles, and, most importantly, they have refrained from trying to stop us as we have worked to make our way in the world. From them, I learned to offer my scholarly critiques from a space of respect and affection—of love—much as they sometimes critiqued my choices and behavior, each in their own style. My mother-in-law was always a great supporter of my work, and it is a matter of great sadness that she could not hold this book in her hands. Little did we know that our summer visit in 2018 would lead to saying our final goodbyes to her, in person and through final rites at our home in Lucknow, nor that her younger brother, our dear Mamaji, would follow her as 2021 began, while we had to remain in the United States due to the COVID-19 pandemic. Least of all did we know that the pandemic would claim two young mothers from our extended family in India in 2021, especially Nishu, who carried her many family responsibilities with grace while continuing to work as a tourism professional.

As the eldest son of the family, Deepak has always assumed that he would have to balance competing roles. He has rolled along with considerable humor through many moves between India and the United States, and within the US, and has made the most of the opportunities created by our strange existence, while dealing with the challenges it has undoubtedly created. Most recently, our daughter, Anushka, has been pulled along. The ease with which she has adjusted to new situations gives us hope for ourselves and for the larger worlds in which we participate.

The years of academic hypermobility that have led me from rural Pennsylvania to the University of South Florida, Bowdoin College, Kenyon College, the University of Notre Dame, the University of Michigan, the University of Virginia, and Lucknow University have broadened my scholarly horizons and inspired me to explore new venues and media for sharing my work. I am endlessly thankful for our expansive families and our networks of friends and colleagues around the world. This book is a small homage to their generosity. For the shortcomings that remain and to anyone whose contributions I have missed, I ask for their pardon, and I humbly request more opportunities to continue our conversations toward greater understanding, remembering and honoring all those who have departed from us along the way.

NOTE ON TRANSLITERATION

WITH NONSPECIALISTS IN MIND AND for the ease of comprehension, I have chosen to use conventional English spellings as commonly used in scholarship and South Asian popular culture for words from South Asian languages that appear in the text and to limit the use of diacritics. For transliteration from Hindi and Urdu scripts, I employ either the US Library of Congress Romanization Tables or spellings in popular usage in South Asia; for example, *Lucknow* rather than *Lakhnau* and *badtameezi* instead of *badtamizi*. The glossary includes pronunciations for key terms.

INFERTILITY IN A
CROWDED COUNTRY

—ᴍ—

INTRODUCTION
Hiding Reproduction

IS THERE ANY LIFE WITHOUT CHILDREN?

If their family members don't say so, outsiders do say so. . . . "Is there any life without children?" If their children have been born too soon, there's trouble. If they've been born after a long time, there's also trouble. And if they haven't been born, there's also trouble.[1]

IN JUNE 2007, DURING A visit to a ramshackle settlement (*basti*) in the old city of Lucknow (Lakhnau), India, a local non-governmental organization (NGO) arranged for me to meet with a group of Muslim women who worked with the organization, which I call Andolan, at their neighborhood office. After introductions, the women shared a little bit about why they were working with Andolan and giving it a home in their neighborhood. They asked about me and what I was studying. Why India? Why this topic? Once they were satisfied, our interaction flowed into conversation about the ways that people think and talk about reproduction, and especially about what women might do when faced with reproductive problems.

In their enthusiasm, several women in that meeting neatly summed up a bind that women often find themselves in, describing

1

the many potential criticisms of their reproductive histories. Children born too soon after marriage, too quickly one after another after marriage, too many of one sex, too few, too delayed, or not at all—each reality could create its own troubles. The trouble, or "disaster" (*museebat*) the women described to me about timing, spacing, sex, or number of children refers to outsiders' views of disordered reproduction. While criticizing unwanted commentary of others (outsiders, *baahar waale*) on reproduction, they also pointed out the surveillance women contend with inside and beyond their own families, whatever their particular reproductive histories.

At a government hospital for women offering infertility treatment, I heard similar sentiments from Hindu, Sikh, and Muslim women. Outsiders commented on women's fertility or lack of fertility, called them names, or asked where daughters-in-law would go, a particular problem if they were attempting to pursue infertility treatment or adoption without letting others in on the details. In the *basti*, hiding reproduction was much more of a challenge than it was for women with more resources to buy privacy, but even then, women would likely be monitored at least until they reached the end of their fertile years. In a country of well over one billion people, and in a state capital city of around three million people, hiding reproduction, and especially hiding novel strategies for procuring children from nosy neighbors and prying family members, requires creativity and practice.

Why hide reproduction? In the United States, contemporary practice shows a proliferation of just the opposite: reproduction proclaimed to the world, even in its earliest stages. In the United States, recent social and technological trends have encouraged people to put their intimate sexual practices on display and have enabled them to detect pregnancy at earlier and earlier stages of gestation and share the results of pregnancy tests with the world. In the United States, many people signal pregnancy by posting the plus signs from pregnancy tests on social media, and as the pregnancy progresses, images of ultrasound examinations and growing "baby bumps" follow, accentuated by tight clothing or bellies bared for the camera. Videos of birth even show up on websites such as YouTube.

Many of these practices appear exotic and shocking to some of the people I have gotten to know over the last twenty years in India. Hiding bodies, traces of sexual activity, and signs of pregnancy whenever possible are practices with high social value across North India. Still, there have been vigorous, long-standing, and ongoing debates about appropriate dress, sexual expression, and fertility within families and at all levels of government for decades, indeed, for centuries. People living in India have been authors of the *Kama Sutra*, purveyors of Victorian prudery, sex workers, and murder victims for choosing their own sexual and life partners. Long histories of colonization and independence, and recent economic, social, and cultural transformations, all play into the ways that people in India understand and manage reproduction.

Sixty percent of the world's population lives in Asia, and the United Nations recently predicted that India will surpass China as the world's most populous country in less than ten years.[2] In this context, across social classes, castes, and religious groups, there are many reasons to hide reproduction. Privilege enables some people to hide more easily than others and may also grant them the ability to flout accepted social practices. While it is young married women whose bodies are subjected to the most intense gaze and the strongest impetus to hide, the implications of concealment extend far beyond them.

Medical anthropologist, physician, and co-founder of Partners in Health Paul Farmer is widely quoted as arguing that "the idea that some lives matter less is the root of all that is wrong with the world."[3] Foreign commentators on India have argued since the nineteenth century, when India had less than one-third of its current population, that India was a crowded country (Ahluwalia 2008; Gupta 2001). These days, few people in India would disagree. I have been told many times, within and outside of India, by Indians and others, that the size of India's population makes life cheap there. My work demonstrates that not all life in India is constructed as equally cheap, and that some lives are indeed very dear. But which lives? To whom are they dear, what do institutional and familial structures tell us about how lives are constructed to matter? How do these structures intersect with emotional dynamics that influence how and how much particular lives matter? How can these structures be transformed toward making a more just reproductive landscape? These are questions at the heart of the reproductive justice movement created and led by women of color in the United States, and questions that Indian people and policymakers have been facing for decades.[4] While activist and advocacy groups such as the New Delhi–based Sama Resource Group for Women and Health (2010, 2012) have been working to ameliorate long-term and urgent reproductive injustices, at the levels of national and international policy and global health, experiences of infertility and reproductive loss have attracted relatively little attention.

In this book, I examine the importance of the concept of *aulad* (aulād)—a culturally specific ideal of biological relatedness between parents and children—for women's lives in North India, particularly when infertility forestalls the expected course of reproduction within marriage. In chapters 1 and 2, I interrogate the construction of the hope for *aulad* alongside ideologies of motherhood in contemporary North India. In chapters 3, 4, and 5, I examine how these ideologies relate to the experiences of women seeking to secure *aulad* through recourse to biomedical infertility treatment, low-cost private health camps, adoption centers, and other private and government resources. The meanings and messages offered by fertile and infertile people and by popular culture illuminate how the categories of children that can and cannot fulfill this ideal are constructed and exemplified by the word *aulad*. The ways people make sense of the meanings of *aulad*, in consort with the structures and discourses they encounter around fertility in daily life, influence how they work to find *aulad*, to approximate *aulad*, and/or to challenge dominant versions of the relationships between children and the families that claim them as their own.

The places and people I sought out in this project reflect my commitment to include minority Muslim women's perspectives on infertility and reproductive loss alongside the voices of people identifying by other religious and social categories. In Lucknow, people's religious backgrounds can usually be guessed by their names, a practice I have used with pseudonyms such as Qudsia baji (*elder sister*, an honorific), Rehana baji, Shabana baji, Dr. Razia, Amina, and so on, referring to Muslim women, and typical Hindu names such as Seema, Rama, Mamta, Manju, and Dr. Kapoor, for Hindu women. Most of the Muslim women who participated in my research were Sunni Muslims. A great deal of historical research on Lucknow has focused on Shi'a Muslims, since the *Nawabs* of Awadh were Shi'as and left a significantly Shi'a impression on Lucknow. However, few women in my study identified themselves as Shi'a.

Anthropologists see human reproduction as a process that is fundamentally cultural. It is sometimes bicultural, combining both biological and cultural elements, and sometimes not, because recognized relationships and identities may not map neatly—or at all—onto relatedness defined through scientific categories of genetics, descent, or other biological notions. Ginsburg and Rapp (1991) followed Emily Martin (1987) and Foucault (1978) in asserting the importance of human reproduction, including fertility, birth, and childcare, as processes of social and cultural renewal. In the contemporary world, they argued that the surveillance and medical control of female bodies are embedded in the practices of development agencies, corporations, and Western medicine. They linked reproduction to the exercise of power within society, emphasizing the power dynamics at work in discourses of population control, access to and choices about new reproductive technologies, and the need to monitor pregnant women (Ginsburg and Rapp 1991, 312, 314–15).

In subsequent work, Ginsburg and Rapp (1995) supported the move to place a stronger emphasis on the political aspects of reproduction, viewing the articulation of state policies regarding fertility as cultural maps of the ideal body politic. In the same volume, Shellee Colen (1995) demonstrated how multiple small and large political, economic, and other policies help hierarchy manifest as stratified reproduction, enabling the reproductive aspirations of some people to take precedence over those of less privileged others. This work has informed a substantial body of research that contributes to theoretical perspectives on kinship and reproduction, the politics of reproduction, and stratified reproduction (Browner and Sargent 2011, Inhorn 2008, Riley 2018), and to rich ethnographic documentation of reproduction around the world. It has also contributed scholarship to related areas such as the examination of reproductive disruption (Inhorn 2007) engendered by diverse interruptions of reproduction from the short term of conception through the long term of the sustainability of families, nations, and other social and cultural groups.

For many anthropologists of reproduction, this body of work serves as one thread of inspiration toward engagement with scholarship and advocacy in the reproductive justice framework, which has continued to develop toward greater expansiveness and inclusivity since its creation in the 1990s (ACRJ 2005; Ross 2006; Ross and Solinger 2017; Ross et al. 2017; Davis 2019; Luna and Luker 2013; Scott 2021). The leading organization with a national and international reach in the United States rooted in this framework is the Atlanta-based SisterSong Women of Color Reproductive Justice Collective. For SisterSong, the fundamentals of reproductive justice are clear: "SisterSong defines Reproductive Justice as the human right to maintain personal bodily autonomy, have children, not have children, and parent the children we have in safe and sustainable communities."[5] A framework that is both theoretical and aimed toward action, it is grounded in the particularities of oppression for marginalized people in the United States, and especially in Black reproductive experiences, broadly conceived. At the same time, the framework emphasizes a broad range of globally intertwined issues that are fundamental to securing human rights and social justice for the vast majority of the world's people.

LOCATING REPRODUCTION: LUCKNOW
IN A CROWDED COUNTRY

Lucknow is the capital city of the state of Uttar Pradesh, in the Gangetic Plains of north-central India. A city with approximately 2.8 million residents as of the 2011 census, Lucknow is the administrative hub of Uttar Pradesh and a focal point for migration for education, employment, and medical treatment. It has only recently been considered for the status of "metro," a city of the first order, a classification long reserved for larger cities such as New Delhi, Mumbai, Kolkata (Calcutta), Chennai (Madras), and Hyderabad. According to the 2011 census, administrative Lucknow overtook industrial Kanpur as the largest city in Uttar Pradesh.[6] Uttar Pradesh continues to be India's most populous state, with about two hundred million residents.[7] In global perspective, if the state of Uttar Pradesh were an independent country, it would be the world's fifth-largest by population (Kopf and Varathan 2017). Large government programs and NGOs center their operations in Uttar Pradesh in Lucknow, and there are several highly regarded educational and medical institutions.

For decades, maternal and infant health, rates of fertility, provisions of birth control, and related matters have focused notable state, national, and international attention on Uttar Pradesh. Large sums of money have been devoted to improving these outcomes. Still, Uttar Pradesh is often singled out as a region of

India that lags behind other Indian states, or is grouped together with other states with poor outcomes, colloquially referred to using the shorthand BIMARU, a clever moniker in Hindi that both refers to the states as "sick" and names the states included.[8] Early in the twenty-first century, popular representations—such as the PBS Nova film *World in the Balance: The People Paradox*— highlighted potential dangers associated with high Indian fertility, particularly in states like Uttar Pradesh, in contrast with the challenges of low fertility in other countries (Holt et al. 2004).[9] International organizations, such as the World Health Organization and United Nations Children's Fund, have operated long-term programs for maternal and child health across India. In Uttar Pradesh, such groups center their operations in Lucknow.

Uttar Pradesh has a relatively high average number of births per woman compared to other states, with a total fertility rate of 2.9, according to the 2018 Sample Registration System (SRS) Statistical Report (all-India 2.2).[10] Uttar Pradesh also accounts for a disproportionate share of maternal and infant mortality among states in India. The Population Reference Bureau puts the current all-India infant mortality rate at thirty-three per one thousand live births.[11] The overall rate has declined appreciably over the years since the start of this project, but there is considerable variation in the rates among regions and classes in India. In Uttar Pradesh, the infant mortality rates appear to be dropping, with 2018 figures at 43/1,000, according to the SRS Statistical Report (all-India in 2018: 32/1,000),[12] down from 83/1,000 in 2000 (all-India in 2000: 68/1,000).[13] Maternal deaths remain among the world's highest, yet they, too, are falling. In Uttar Pradesh, deaths have officially declined from 292 for every 100,000 live births in 2010–12 to 197 deaths per 100,000 live births in 2016–18, yet these numbers were and remain higher than the all-India average of 178 per 100,000 births in 2010–12 and 113 in 2016–18.[14] Infertility as an aspect of reproductive health has, until recently, received very little attention from such agencies, and has been difficult

to track statistically, although medical and spiritual professionals offering solutions for infertility, as well biomedical and other
medical systems offering treatment, have flourished. Behind and
beyond the statistics lie, in the case of any reproductive indicator,
a more detailed picture to be found by breaking down statistics
by urban or rural residence, caste, class, or religion and through
narrative accounts of embodied experiences, births, deaths, and
desires fulfilled and unfulfilled, and through an examination of
the cultural ideologies that can influence desires and actions.

Histories of the last two and a half centuries weave through
the demographic, political, cultural, and structural composition
of Lucknow. It is the heart of the Awadh region of central/east-
ern Uttar Pradesh, which has long been proclaimed to embrace
a "mixed culture/manner" (*Ganga-Yamuni tehzeeb*). The eigh-
teenth- and nineteenth-century rulers of Awadh were known as
Nawabs, Shi'a Muslim rulers whose traces remain in Lucknow,
despite the large-scale destruction of the 1857 Rebellion (otherwise known as the Sepoy Mutiny) in North India. The *Nawabs*
famously sponsored the construction of Hindu temples and a variety of Muslim religious structures in proximity to one another,
among other policies directed toward keeping the peace among
the inhabitants (Llewellyn-Jones 1985).

The cultivation of peaceful interaction among religious communities during the *Nawabi* period has been memorialized—and
sometimes idealized—not only in the architectural heritage of
Lucknow but also in films such as Satyajit Ray's *Shatranj ke Khilari*
(*The Chess Players*)[15] and in the poetry of rulers of Awadh such as
the last *Nawab*, Wajid 'Ali Shah. Wajid 'Ali Shah composed Urdu
couplets about the Lucknow region such as *"Hum ishq ke bande
hain mazhab se nahin vaqif / Gar kaaba hua to kya butkhana hua
to kya."* In less poetic English, his sentiment remains: "We are the
votaries of Love and unacquainted with religion / To us it does
not matter, whether it is *kaba* or a temple."[16] Such sentiments have
been embraced by people in Lucknow who assert the unity of

God, regardless of the name one uses (such as Ram or Rahim, references to a Hindu deity and a Sufi word for God, "the merciful"). They have also been challenged many times through regional and national politics and through conflicts between Shi'a and Sunni Muslims. As an Indian city, Lucknow has historically had a low incidence of violent conflicts between Hindus and Muslims, which have been more prominent and disruptive in other parts of India in recent decades. Political scientist Ashutosh Varshney (2002) argues that the high degree of integration of members of different religious communities in economic pursuits such as the *chikan* embroidery industry, coupled with the cleavage between Shi'a and Sunni Muslims, largely account for the high degree of communal peace in Lucknow at the mass level, everyday interactions among elites notwithstanding (171, 175–78).

Many scholars argue that the full British takeover of Awadh in 1856 spurred the rebellion against British rule that engulfed North India the following year (Fisher 1993; Mukherjee 1984). The annexation began a long process of remaking Lucknow that has continued since Indian independence from colonial rule in 1947, as newer residents and leaders create their own marks on the physical and cultural landscape of the city. Lucknow is the present capital city and administrative hub of the state of Uttar Pradesh. Lucknow is also the seat of power for the chief minister (equivalent to a governor in the United States). Since *Nawabi* times, Lucknow has expanded considerably to accommodate the construction projects of various rulers and new residents, mostly from other parts of Uttar Pradesh, although the older parts of the city still form a dense, vibrant urban core. By way of its history and heritage, Lucknow is particularly important as a center both of Muslim population (Sunni and Shi'a) and of institutes of Islamic learning in Uttar Pradesh. Large medical institutes with teaching faculties and clinical practice attract patients from the smaller cities, towns, and villages surrounding Lucknow, and public and private practitioners of biomedical ("Western"

or "English"), Ayurvedic, and Unani systems of medicine are in
abundant supply throughout the city. Although the capital of a
state that still takes population growth to be a major policy issue,
Lucknow at the time of my field research was home to over half
a dozen private fertility clinics in addition to government clinics
that offer both infertility treatment services and birth control.
In common parlance, birth control alone is usually what people
mean when they talk about family planning.

People identifying as Hindus, Muslims, Sikhs, Christians,
and members of other religious groups reside in contemporary
Lucknow. Their presence can be felt in the built environment of
temples (mandirs), mosques and other Muslim holy places (mas-
jids, imambaras, mazaars, dargahs), Sikh gurudwaras, and Christian churches, and in the flow of everyday life, even as people
embrace or reject personal religious practice. This mingling and
separation varies greatly depending on which part of the city
forms the base of reference. By and large, people claiming these
various religious identities have tolerated one another peacefully,
and have sometimes taken delight in their diverse holidays and
traditions. Friendship between people from diverse religious and
caste backgrounds has been common, and, although not without occasional tension and conflict, it deeply impacts conduct in
everyday life. The history of proclamations about the mixed culture of Lucknow and the harmony among its people serve as an
important ideological touchpoint for this project. For example,
women from different backgrounds argued with great conviction
that dealing with reproductive absence and loss was so difficult
and important that women would be quite willing to cross cultural and religious boundaries in search of a child. The openness
of access to religious buildings in Lucknow, such as churches,
Hindu temples, imambaras (imāmbāṛā; buildings in which the
relics used during Muslim Muharram observances are stored),
and the graves of Sufi Muslim saints and other holy people
(dargahs or mazaars) contributed to these impressions and the

possibility for women to pursue help from many locations. I heard over and again, especially by people with no personal history of infertility, that religious identity would not be a deterrent to pursuing treatment or healing. Many women would readily visit holy places associated with any faith, so long as that place had a reputation for healing.

Yet, I also found strong indications of divisions among women's abilities to pursue particular strategies for obtaining children. Many of these boundaries revolved around aspects of religious belief or practice and aspects of financial constraint. People stressed to me the common stigma and distress faced by women dealing with a lack of children, regardless of religious identity. I demonstrate similarities and distinctions that can be traced to Indian government regulations, the interpretation of religious law, and everyday interactions among government employees, activists, and medical practitioners with people seeking children.

While many women in Lucknow stressed the victimization of women whose fertility had failed the expectations of "society" (*samaj*, samāj) and of their marital families, I found myself often surprised and impressed by the resilience of people with whom I worked. Those I interviewed in clinics were still actively seeking to overcome infertility, and most maintained optimism about their chances. Some women mingled their stories of adversity and failure with their sense of accomplishment in pursuing treatment or in success in other areas of their lives. Although their stories were sometimes difficult to listen to, this was not so in an unmitigated, unrelenting sense; despair, hope, and realism were often mixed together in women's accounts. My research points to many of the unique difficulties faced by Muslim women, among women in India—but I have cautioned myself, and I caution readers, not to see this as another story about brown women who need to be rescued by white men (Spivak 1988) or women, or about Muslim women in special need of rescue by the West (Abu-Lughod 2013, 2002). Throughout my research, I met

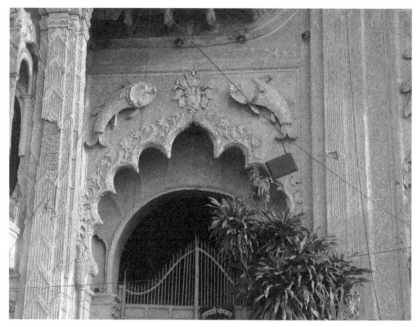

Figure b.1. Built heritage of eighteenth- and nineteenth-century Nawabi Awadh, exemplified by fish and style of brick and stucco work, Qaiserbagh, Lucknow. (Photo by author.)

extremely articulate, self-possessed, and self-confident women from different religious, caste, and class backgrounds, including Muslim women. In many cases, they were much more articulate, self-possessed, and self-confident than the researcher learning about their lives.

Muslim women I met in Lucknow often defied stereotypes of "Islamic women" that circulate in the United States. Education, class, and family expectations about religious observance count to an enormous extent in shaping the agency Muslim women are able to assert, similar to other Indian women. This may be true even while observing fairly rigorous separation of the sexes (purdah, pardā), as Zoya Hasan and Ritu Menon (2005) demonstrate in their collection on the diversity of Muslim women's lives in India.[17] While Islamic and Indian law have historically narrowed the options for Muslim women to obtain children, the Quran offers comfort to those who live without children in a passage that was quoted to me on several occasions: "So He leaves barren who He wills" (42:50). And yet, as an account set in public and semipublic spaces in contemporary Lucknow, this is not a story exclusively about Muslim women.

Some of the architectural remnants of the period of *Nawabi* rule in Lucknow have been restored by local trusts or government programs. Most crumble away a bit more with each passing year, physical legacies of Shi'a Muslim, then British colonial, preeminence and authority. They serve as reminders of pasts that are being swept away by development and by successive state government leaders who seek to draw attention to the heroes of their own political parties. The physical environment of Lucknow visualizes postcolonial struggles over identity and belonging, as shifting demographics and political currents have left their traces on the city. Yet the older legacies linger in some of the most well-established clinical spaces, housed in grand, but not fashionable, British colonial-era buildings that evoke the prestige of their connection to the power of the colonial era, English language, and biomedical science. Their high ceilings and thick walls confound efforts to maintain clean, sterile spaces within, and necessitate continual retrofitting to meet the requirements of particular procedures. The congestion and barely contained chaos of the old city outside often seem to make their way inside, with the bustle of patients, visitors, and staff, and the gathering of dust and frequent disturbances of power and water supply.

The two hospitals where I conducted most of my clinical interviews and observations were established during the British colonial era in Lucknow. Their architecture and the names people in Lucknow used to refer to them marked this heritage, even though the official names tended to change with party control of state government, as part of efforts to indigenize government institutions. Historical and demographic perspectives on fertility and population in India reverberate in health provision not only through physical spaces but also through the social, cultural, and historical categories and reference points medical staff and patients brought with them. From the outside, large-scale demographic data tend to render infertility and people suffering from it invisible and, perhaps, unimaginable (Fledderjohann and Barnes 2018), at the same time that they may be rendered hypervisible in state and national discourse as presumed contributors to high fertility.

THE FERTILITY-INFERTILITY DIALECTIC AND REPRODUCTIVE POLITICS

Frank van Balen and Marcia Inhorn (2002) have emphasized the importance of examining infertility in areas of the world where state reproductive health programs have mainly focused on reducing the number of births. In their edited volume on infertility in global perspective, they argue that

> focusing on infertility in "overpopulated" areas of the world reveals much about the "fertility-infertility dialectic" (Inhorn 1994, p. 23) or the relationship of tension and contrast that exists between fertility and infertility on both the microsociological level of individual human experience and the macrosociological level of reproductive politics. . . . The very existence of infertility in high-fertility regimes represents a challenge to monolithic assumptions about the nature of population control and the extent to which fertility-control orthodoxies are in fact resisted and reconfigured in practice, particularly in non-Western populations among whom infertility is demographically significant and greatly feared. (van Balen and Inhorn 2002, 7)

During my time in Lucknow, I found that the macro level of reproductive politics rarely figured prominently in individual expressions of child desire. That is, I did not hear women saying that they wanted to have larger families to win a national demographic war. Women across the social spectrum who had not personally experienced infertility problems dismissed the importance of religion or caste background with reference to the suffering associated with infertility, for example, and asserted that in cases of infertility, women disregard religious boundaries in pursuit of a solution to their problem. However, political issues of religion and identity did come into play when women, whether or not they had personal histories of dealing with infertility, spoke about approaching healthcare professionals for assistance. They often expressed worries about discrimination based on religion and economic status. Structurally, "family planning" in India has mostly focused on the provision of birth control for birth spacing and fertility limitation (compare with Bledsoe 2002). Yet, people seeking to alleviate their childless state have also approached family-planning workers for assistance in expanding their families. This task has received much less attention and funding in government-run programs than efforts to reduce fertility.

Between the micro level of human experience and the macro level of politics identified by van Balen and Inhorn (2002), the familial politics of in/fertility, akin to what Jan Brunson (2016) refers to in her work on Nepal as "projects of reproduction," contingent and temporally extended (113), emerged as a major focus of talk about reproduction in Lucknow. In this middle space, the implications of fertility, as Sudhir Kakar (1978) has suggested, affect not only the psychological profile of men and women of reproductive age but also the relationships between family members that are both personal and political. Families in Uttar Pradesh encourage their married children to reproduce, although they generally do not dwell on the particulars about how to become parents and tend to avoid overt references to sexuality. They make their wishes known in roundabout ways and may continue to do so even after the successful birth of a child with hints such as "he's lonely . . . he needs a sister . . . she needs a companion" or "just one more and you'll be done." The extent to which family members and other acquaintances advocate continued fertility also depends on the particular social context of the individual. For example, in some families the idea that two sons are necessary to ensure the survival of at least one still holds sway (Holt et al. 2004). Others express less qualified reproductive standards. As one Hindu woman told me, "after two, no one will ask you to have a third." Many people have adopted the small family norm but have not given up on the importance of sons, and demographic trends continue to reflect interventions that lead to a population with more boys than girls. Limits to the support of families for continued fertility do exist, and in some social contexts, giving birth to "too many" children can also lead to censure from other family members, even if continued fertility is due to the pursuit of sons. Building on the infertility-fertility dialectic and related scholarship, there are new calls for an integration of social-science research in fertility and infertility through expanded collaborations across disciplines (Riley and Brunson 2018) or, more specifically, through a "reproductive career" approach (Johnson et al. 2018). These approaches aim to bring together perspectives from anthropology, sociology, and demography not only to include infertility where it has too often been left out (Riley and McCarthy 2003; Singh 2018) but also to account for changes over the life course, recognizing and looking more deeply into the connections between fertility and infertility in individual lives, understanding how they are interwoven in cultural norms, and examining how relationships between fertility and infertility can matter for reproductive health and policy decisions.

In India and around the world, the politics of reproduction often influence the reproductive lives of people living within states with explicit or implicit priorities pertaining to the shape of the body politic (Ginsburg and Rapp 1991).[18] Since independence in 1947, the Indian state has continued the British colonial practice of administering family (or personal) law according to established customs of different religious groups to protect minority rights in matters of marriage, divorce, adoption, and inheritance. Fulfilling the promise of equal rights for all citizens in democratic India, while dealing with the diversity of India's population, has presented a long-term challenge. Michel Foucault (1978) identified population control as a key expression of sovereign biopower, especially through the use of demography, public health, and other hygienic "civic services" to implement discipline among citizens (135, 139–40). State interest in sexual affairs functions to discipline bodies and regulate populations and define national citizenship (145). Kalpana Ram (2001, 84) argues that planners, demographers, and policymakers in India have equated the state vision of reproduction and fertility—"small family, happy family" and "we two, our two"—with modern rationality, relegating those with other opinions to the degraded position of "premodern." Medical professionals often considered women, especially those living in rural areas, too ignorant to follow birth-control regimens closely, and so they focused on irreversible (or difficult to reverse) methods of birth control like sterilization (Jolly 2001, 22; Ram 2001, 91, 94). The use of coercion in controlling births, particularly for people whose fertility has been stigmatized and who are seen by political and/or medical authorities as less likely to voluntarily reduce their fertility, is certainly not limited to the Indian subcontinent, as Dorothy Roberts (1997) has argued with respect to African American fertility in the particular context of the United States.

Ram (2001) asserts that those groups categorized as "premodern" in their reproductive consciousness are the same groups that become configured as "Other" in citizenship, especially Indian Muslims (111–12). Islamic leaders in India have been most vocal in objecting to sterilization on religious grounds, asserting that acting to prevent God's will to bring a new soul into the world is sinful (Khan 1979, 172). While Muslims express a variety of opinions on this subject, many agree in their objection to

terminal methods of fertility control, such as the male and female sterilization government programs strongly encourage.
Across religious boundaries, people have cited infant and child
mortality—the likelihood of loss—as an important reason for
rejecting irreversible forms of birth control (Pinto 2003, 419; Jeffery and Jeffery 1997, 104).

While national-level politics about the religious composition
of the nation-state have echoes in the fertility decisions expressed
by women in my research, I found these dynamics to be muted.
They were most relevant when I explained my research project
to people I encountered in the field, especially when I mentioned
that I was particularly interested in *Muslim* women's experiences
of dealing with infertility. That idea sometimes provoked confusion. One Muslim professor of literature at Lucknow University
initially turned my research completely around as he tried to
explain to me that I *must* surely be interested in how many children Muslim families in the old city have because I would undoubtedly find families there with ten or twelve children. When
I pressed that my interest was actually in women who either did
not have children or had encountered problems in conceiving
or giving birth to live children, it gave him pause. What perhaps
seemed like an expected and conventional project from a foreign
scholar turned out not to be quite so. Yet, it did not stop him from
giving me several useful recommendations about people to meet
for help with finding contacts for my research.

In conversations with acquaintances who were not directly
involved in my research, I often gave a very brief description of
my interests. If I mentioned my particular interest in infertility
among Muslims, that detail often surprised non-Muslims. Some
people scoffed at the idea that there might be Muslims suffering from a lack of children, since they were more familiar with
the stereotypes of large Muslim families. Others thought that
if there were Muslims suffering from infertility, this was a good

thing, since India was already overpopulated, particularly with Muslims. So, if Muslims were unable to have children, this would be good for India.

Prejudices about the fertility of particular groups defined by religion (and, to a lesser extent, by caste and economic status) have been part of national public discourse in India for well over a hundred years, as Sanjam Ahluwalia (2008), Charu Gupta (2001), and Patricia Jeffery and Roger Jeffery (2006), among others, document. These categories have extended into demography, as exemplified by Joshi et al. (2003) and others. From the perspective of national politics, it seems reasonable to read the politics of fertility as tending toward reproductive competition between large groups, mainly Hindus and Muslims or, to a lesser extent, Christians and Dalits. Simply put, more children may tilt the balance of power by increasing their numbers. Even in this discourse, however, there are dissenting voices, such as the prominent Lucknow-based Shi'a cleric Maulana Kalbe Sadiq, who publicly argued for a "quality over quantity" mode of reproduction.[19] In other words, he urged Muslims to have only as many children as they could support and educate well to compete for jobs and in business, rather than to press for power purely through the expansion of their numbers.[20] Dr. Sadiq, who held a PhD in Arabic from Lucknow University, made this argument numerous times, including in a lecture that I attended at the Shah Najaf Imambara in Lucknow in December 2006.

The Prevalence and Relevance of Infertility in India

Although Indian fertility and reproduction have long been subjects of intense study and intervention through programs run by government organizations and NGOs, Indian infertility has rarely figured significantly as a topic for close analysis. While indicating the inadequacy of substantial research on this aspect of reproductive health in India, Shireen Jejeebhoy (1998), an India-based demographer working with the Population Council in New

Delhi, estimated in the late 1990s that approximately 10 percent of couples in South Asia suffer from infertility at some point in their reproductive years, similar to the rates in other areas of the world (17). She made the case that infertility had been examined mostly as an incidental sideline in studies on high fertility in South Asia and called for more detailed research on infertility in South Asia. More recent demographic work suggests that at least eighteen million couples in India may be affected by infertility (Ganguly and Unisa 2010).

Over the last decade and more, the practice of transnational gestational surrogacy—otherwise dubbed "wombs for rent"—has drawn media attention within India to the biomedical infertility sector. The many legal and cultural complexities associated with surrogacy have generated a flowering of work by journalists, filmmakers, and social scientists on infertility treatment in India, focused on the ways that fertile Indian women's bodies became the commodified vessels through which people from other countries fulfilled their desires for children (Deomampo 2016; Majumdar 2018; Pande 2014; Rudrappa 2015; Saravanan 2018; Singh 2014, 2018; Vora 2015). Yet, the persistent issues relating to how women living in India understand and deal with their own infertility and struggle to create and sustain families have not yet received that level of attention.

Defining and Locating Infertility: Plurality by Perspective

Definitions of infertility vary among cultures, even where biomedicine has a strong presence, and a wide variety of methods for offering the hope of biological children have a long history in cross-cultural perspectives, from ethnomedical and herbal remedies to massage and spiritual intervention. Theories of procreation in particular cultural contexts underpin the meanings of infertility and may influence perceptions of who is responsible for the creative act in conception, and who is responsible for the failure to conceive. For example, as Carol Delaney (1991) argues in her work on rural Turkish theories of coming-into-being, agricultural metaphors of the seed and the field attribute the child's being to the male contribution, while portraying the female role as one of receiving and nurturing (8, 12). In this monogenetic (one-source, descent through one parent) system, paternity is about exclusively creating a child's essence, begetting. Maternity pertains to its nurturance, bearing (Delaney 1986, 494–95). However, cases of infertility are usually viewed not as a lack of potency of the seed but as the rejection of the seed by the field (Delaney 1991, 52).

With reference to India, anthropologist R. S. Khare (1996) has argued that "human diseases have closely interrelated physical, natural, bodily, social, and moral and supernatural causes, expressions, and consequences. They do not concern only the physical body or some of its parts" (843). This multiplicity, common in India's medically plural environment, is also characteristic of infertility, even though the status of infertility as a "disease" is a point on which social scientists and medical specialists often differ. Biomedical definitions of infertility vary but tend to focus on the inability of a couple to conceive after between six and twenty-four months of unprotected intercourse. These states can be further divided into primary infertility/sterility—complete inability to conceive—and secondary infertility, inability to conceive after previous pregnancy.

Even in the most medicalized situations, cultural understandings of infertility are not absent. Patients' experiences of treatment suffuse their own interpretations of infertility, the relationships that impinge on their seeking treatment, and their ability and/or willingness to follow the treatments recommended by physicians and other medical staff. Definitions of infertility from particular local perspectives often indicate reproductive ideals by pointing out the "failure" of a couple to achieve them; for example, the inability to produce a son or inability to produce the culturally ideal number of children. In Hindi/Urdu, the term *banjhpan* (bānjhpan) most commonly refers to the state of in-fertility, but its closest meaning is *sterile*. Both a woman (but not a man) and an agricultural field can be *banjh* (bānjh, barren). Indigenous categories used to define infertility should be inves-tigated in particular cultural contexts, rather than assumed to be a universally recognizable medical condition. Local definitions, theories about the body, procreation, sources of disease, and re-productive difficulties build the context within which infertility becomes meaningful.

Biomedicine has developed numerous diagnostic tests for de-termining the causes of infertility rooted in the individual body, yet some cases fall outside of biomedicine's diagnostic capability. Many South Asians visit several types of specialists either simul-taneously or one after the other in search of healing (Unisa 1999). Physician Veena Mulgaonkar's (2001) study of infertility among Mumbai slum-dwellers indicates that poor childless couples at-tribute infertility to numerous sources, ranging from improper food consumption and reproductive tract or sexual disorders, to supernatural causes and the breach of cultural norms (147). These diverse explanatory models about infertility suggest multiple strategies for the alleviation of childlessness, including medical, ritual, and social interventions.

Choices of particular healers are sometimes influenced by re-ligious preferences, but not universally. Hindus very often seek healing at sites associated with Muslim holy people at shrines or with living Muslim healers. Intermingling healing strategies is part of the common *Ganga-Yamuni* mixed cultural ethos in North India.[21] However, anecdotal evidence suggests that Muslims are less likely to engage in these multiple strategies. When they cross religious boundaries, such strategies are more likely to garner criticism by Muslim religious and social leaders than by leaders of other religious communities because of the danger of violating Islam's principle of the unity of God, and because of the politics of Muslim identity in South Asia.

Interpreting and Addressing the Absence of Children

Involuntary childlessness should be distinguished from the "childfree living" advocated by some infertile couples, potentially fertile couples, and others who accept and/or embrace life without children. Adult life without children finds little acceptance in most of the world, including places such as India, where pronatal cultural sentiments intersect and sometimes conflict with efforts by national government organizations and numerous NGOs to promote small families. Women's narratives of infertility and involuntary childlessness (overview in Inhorn 2008; also especially Riessman 2002; Inhorn 1994) demonstrate that culturally specific ideas about what constitutes legitimate kinship ties, gender roles, and status shape the significance of infertility and involuntary childlessness (van Balen and Inhorn 2002, 11).

The use of biomedical treatments including assisted reproductive technologies (ARTs) such as in vitro fertilization (IVF, otherwise known in India as "test-tube baby") and intracytoplasmic sperm injection (a specialized form of IVF in which a single sperm is directly injected into an ovum through micromanipulation) is one potential method of alleviating involuntary childlessness that may result from infertility, but there are many others. Adoption, temporary fosterage, and, for some, the acquisition of pets may also resolve the problem of involuntary childlessness, but all of these strategies need to be examined in the particular context in which they may be undertaken, rather than offered up as universal solutions to the "problems" associated with infertility.

New technological means of controlling and enhancing fertility have both created avenues for innovation in procreation—"strategic" naturalization of particular relationships (Thompson 2001) and selective interpretation of religious texts to regulate the use of ARTs (Kahn 2000)—and strengthened existing reproductive ideals (Das Gupta 1987) around the world. Although Muslims in other countries do use ARTs as one means of overcoming involuntary childlessness, and specialists in Islamic law and ethics have offered legal opinions on the appropriate use of these technologies (Sachedina 2009; Inhorn 2003; Anees 1989), Muslims were largely absent from the biomedical infertility clinics in major Indian cities (New Delhi, Mumbai [Bombay], Jaipur) studied separately by Aditya Bharadwaj and Anjali Widge in the late 1990s (Bharadwaj 2001, 53; Widge 2005, 228).

Patricia Jeffery and Roger Jeffery (1997, 223) assert that Muslims in India are comparatively less educated and poorer than Hindus, and that these factors must be crucial considerations in analyses of reproduction in India. Their particular emphasis echoes Faye Ginsburg and Rayna Rapp's (1991, 315) argument that studies of infertility must include analysis of how economics impact the management of infertility in particular communities. To the extent possible based on available data, I draw attention to the convergence and divergence of reproductive ideologies and strategies for dealing with the absence of children among Lucknow's diverse population. The chapters that follow document women's perspectives across diverse religious and caste backgrounds, including their assertions of infertile women's common experiences and strategies regardless of religious background, while directing attention to the unique challenges that Muslim women encounter in seeking children. I highlight similarities and distinctions that can be traced to Indian government regulations, the interpretation of Islamic law, and everyday interactions among government employees, activists, and medical practitioners with people seeking children.

METHODS: RESEARCHING REPRODUCTION IN INDIA

This book draws on interviews and participant observation conducted during sixteen months of ethnographic field research on fertility and infertility experiences in Lucknow, Uttar Pradesh, between 2005 and 2007 and during a short return research period in 2015–16. Throughout the research period, I met with, interviewed, and attended events sponsored by academics, medical professionals, and social activists working on issues relating to gender, poverty, and power in Lucknow. These interactions inform the context of interpretation for other sources examined here, which are also grounded in long-term study and research in India spanning over four years since 1998. I have also been part of a transnational family moving between Lucknow and the United States since 2002. These experiences inform my writing and my understandings of the city, and of the contexts of family and fertility in India.

I conducted semistructured interviews with more than fifty women from a variety of religious, class, and caste backgrounds who were suffering from infertility. Interviews took place in government infertility clinics and outside of clinical spaces, and participants were recruited opportunistically rather than through a purposeful structured sample. Members of several local NGOs assisted with recruiting participants outside of clinics. In addition, I observed the work of fifteen doctors specializing in gynecology and women's health across public and private clinics, and the work of other medical staff members, with whom I conducted structured interviews and more informal interactions during clinic hours. Few potential respondents, selected on the basis of their attendance at the clinic or through reference by leaders of one of several NGOs, declined to participate. However, interview time in clinical spaces was limited by interruptions caused by scheduled procedures. I conducted all interviews myself, drawing informally from an interview guide and allowing the conversations to take shape according to women's preferences and responses. To protect confidentiality, interviews with patients in infertility clinics were recorded by hand. Other interviews were audiotaped. I explained the research to each participant and obtained and documented oral consent from each participant using procedures approved by the Institutional Review Boards at the University of Virginia, and later at the University of Michigan. Interviews took place in the Hindi and Urdu vernacular language common to Uttar Pradesh, and occasionally in English, according to the preferences of participants. I am fluent in Hindi and Urdu and have become familiar with local colloquial languages through years of formal language study and residence in Uttar Pradesh and neighboring Bihar State, so I did not work with a translator for any of the interviews. My data also come from newspapers, research produced by the government of India, and Hindi and Urdu films and literature. The University of Virginia, the University of Michigan, the American Institute of Indian Studies, and the Eunice Kennedy Shriver National Institute of Child Health and Human Development (through a Center Grant [R24 HD041028]), a postdoctoral training grant to the University of Michigan's Population Studies Center (T32 HD007339), and a Mellon Foundation postdoctoral teaching grant to Bowdoin College provided funding for preliminary, secondary, and field research and support for access to library, administrative, and mentoring resources throughout the writing process. Lucknow University provided research affiliation and intellectual community during field research. The ultimate decisions about study design, data collection, analysis, and interpretation, and decisions about writing and publication have been mine. I translated and analyzed field notes, audio recordings, and available documentation, and data gathered through interviews, observation, and participant observation. Outside of biomedical infertility clinics, respondents were recruited through referrals from friends, relatives, or social workers in NGOs, giving attention to including participants from diverse local backgrounds to the greatest extent possible. In biomedical infertility clinics, women presenting themselves for treatment were interviewed apart from any accompanying individuals while they waited for an examination. Some interviews were conducted over several visits to the clinic for continued treatment. Medical staff in clinics provided contextual information and assisted with recruitment of participants, but staff members were usually not present during interviews. Women were informed in consent procedures that their participation was voluntary and that agreeing or declining to participate in the research would not affect their treatment at the clinic. The vast majority of women recruited in clinics eagerly agreed to share their experiences. The data presented here do not include patient interviews conducted in private infertility clinics (see Bharadwaj 2016; Unisa 1999; Widge 2001, 2005). I focus instead on services provided through clinics in public sector (government) hospitals, which have received less scholarly attention and have begun to offer a wide range of infertility services as part of their reproductive health program more recently, at much lower prices than in the private sector.

At the time of the first field research, I was a childfree doctoral candidate from the United States in my late twenties. Many women with whom I interacted asked probing questions to determine these details of my status relative to their situations, and their comments often included admonishments to try for children soon. I reflect on these dynamics and their implications for the research in more detail below and elsewhere (Singh 2016). I also draw on scholarly, popular media, and literary perspectives on kinship and the use of ARTs in India to analyze continuity and change in representations of reproduction.

The cooperation of medical staff was crucial to that part of the field research. Even though hospitals could be crowded and women were often in a hurry, this was the easiest place to locate and talk with women suffering from infertility. Women entered the treatment area on their own, away from the prying eyes of neighbors and relatives, and they were in a space where others were experiencing similar problems. Would women really answer the intimate questions that I would ask? In this space, most talked freely about their histories of treatment and of dealing with infertility on an everyday basis. Indeed, many seemed pleased to talk with me. However, that interest yielded only a very small number of invitations to come to their homes and talk further: the clinic was a place where the ability to maintain secrecy and confidentiality was relatively assured. Initial interviews in clinics usually lasted for forty-five to sixty minutes, and I met some women multiple times because their visits to the clinic coincided with mine. I interviewed all women who were willing to participate, unless the head nurse advised me to leave someone alone. She served both as a gatekeeper and as an extra ethical buffer in the hospital setting, but only in a few cases did she indicate to me that the person involved was particularly troubled or traumatized by what they had gone through. I trusted that the nurse judged them too sensitive to be comfortable expressing their views.

In the hospitals where I worked, men waited outside the infertility unit (a public space), while their partners waited inside (a relatively private place). The NGOs that helped facilitate my research outside of hospitals catered exclusively to women and children, most of them Muslims who observed greater and lesser degrees of separation of the sexes. To a great extent, it was the *absence* of men that gave me the opportunity to talk frankly with women about their experiences with infertility. Bharadwaj's (2016) work provides insight into the views of men as part of couples in big-city infertility clinics in the 1990s, and more work remains to be done specifically on men's perspectives on infertility and reproductive loss in India.

Other published work on the social dynamics of infertility in India has focused mainly or exclusively on people receiving treatment in private biomedical clinics (Bharadwaj 2003, 2016; Widge 2001) or through an NGO (Mulgaonkar 2001). Both Bharadwaj (2016, 2003, 2001) and Widge (2005, 2001) noted that all of the people who participated in their studies were Hindus. In building on this work in the anthropology of reproduction, I sought a wider frame than the clinical one and a greater diversity of experiential perspectives, which led me to focus deeply on one city and to seek Muslim perspectives as an integral part of my work. In Lucknow, I certainly did not find that only Hindus suffered from infertility, contrary to what some non-Muslims told me (i.e., that all Muslims have ten children). I began my research outside of clinics and only began conducting interviews in infertility clinics when I had gained a significant understanding of the broader social context in which women experience infertility and childlessness in Lucknow. This strategy helped me to document perspectives from a wider range of people and also to situate reproductive woes that did not begin and end with visits to biomedical clinics within their local moral worlds (Kleinman 1999).

Searching for women who either were currently suffering from infertility or had suffered from it in the past outside of the clinic was a challenging prospect. This was true partly because of their relatively small numbers in a city of millions, but more so because of the secrecy involved in infertility and the embarrassment felt by others about asking a friend, acquaintance, or relative to share their stories. In the process of searching, though, I heard from people who had not gone through infertility themselves but were eager to share their perspectives. As they talked about society; what "people think" (*log sochte hain ki*); and the experiences of others they knew regarding infertility, adoption, the importance of sons, and the meanings of children; I learned about the social contexts within which women dealing with infertility decide how to negotiate the local resources available to them. Across a variety of settings in Lucknow, from school and college campuses to meetings of NGOs and women's social organizations, in homes, in shopping malls, and in local physicians' offices, it became clear that even if women were secret about their individual histories, there were broad social conversations and shared expectations about people suffering because of infertility. These conversations helped illuminate the social context of reproductive disruption— infertility and reproductive absences and losses—in Lucknow.

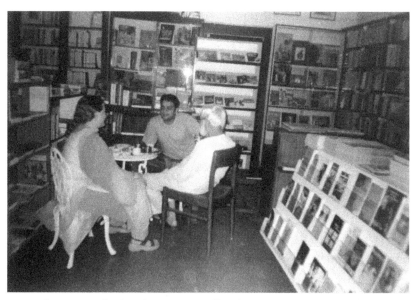

Figure b.2. One of many discussions of books, culture, history, and life over tea with Mr. Ram Advani (in white) inside Ram Advani Booksellers, Hazratganj, Lucknow. (Photo by author.)

This ethnography engages ideologies and experiences of reproductive loss and social stigma, based on perspectives from women from across the social spectrum in class, caste, and religious background. It also includes representations of reproduction from broader public culture: medical personnel, newspaper reporters, Hindi/Urdu writers, and filmmakers. These contributions address the nature of reproduction, the importance of particular ideals of biological relatedness, and the possibility of adopting children. These types of representations circulate widely in India and form an important part of how people frame their understandings of infertility and the resultant absence of children. They demonstrate how crucial cultural context, including popular culture and media, is to understanding what fertility means—and the implications of reproductive absence and loss for the people experiencing these disruptions within their own local moral worlds (Kleinman 1999). As the long-term effects of the COVID-19 pandemic and interlocking environmental and social crises reverberate around the world, the vulnerability of the systems that might care for us—from kin networks to healthcare to national and international governance—has been made newly visible to some, and more plain and visceral to others. The disruption wrought by this time offers the world an opportunity to imagine anew how we create, ignore, and destroy bonds with one another.

ETHNOGRAPHIC ENTWINEMENTS

The most moving and memorable ethnographies that have shaped my own scholarship have been works that take very seriously calls from anthropology (Bateson 2012, 1989; Khare 1992) and feminist studies (Haraway 1988) for nuanced consideration of how researchers' personal histories shape the knowledge they generate at every stage of the research and writing process. Researchers all have particular positions in relation to the human beings from whom and with whom they learn—whether it be with or against them (or both)—and whether they are called informants, participants, interlocutors, friends, enemies, or something else. Scholars who do interweave an evaluation of the researcher's "I" meaningfully into their ethnography (Behar 1996; Khare 2011; Layne 2003; Pinto 2008; Rapp 1999) have been "moral pioneers" (Rapp 1999) themselves in acknowledging their intimate relations with the people and/or topic they study. They have tackled the special advantages, challenges, pain, and frustration presented by those entwinements, and encouraged new generations of scholars to follow their model and answer Edith Turner's (2007) call for inclusion and validation of ethnographers' own experiences in their role as coproducers of a humanistic anthropology (110). Feminist scholars, Dalit writers, and others who have seen themselves as occupying marginal social locations have historically taken their positioning rather more seriously than other producers of knowledge and have pressed others most convincingly to do so.

In the anthropology of reproduction, a specific area of cultural and medical anthropology, positionality often emerges as a crucial part of the story, as scholars have revealed the extremely intimate, personal, and traumatic events that have led them to conduct research on a particular subject. For example, Rapp's (1999) work on amniocentesis and selective abortion found its genesis in her own history of prenatal diagnosis of Down's syndrome that led her to terminate the pregnancy. Layne (2003) used excruciating, even gruesome detail to describe her work on pregnancy loss that was rooted in her own experience of seven pregnancy losses ("miscarriages") and other reproductive difficulties. Davis (2019) drew on her own reproductive history to ground her examination of Black families' journeys through reproductive risks in the United States. These scholars, and others who take similar approaches, have acknowledged their intimate entwinements with their research subject and tackled the special advantages, challenges, pain, and frustration presented by them.

When I was preparing for fieldwork, the seeming advantages of such entwinements led others in my PhD cohort to suggest (in jest) that I should tell people that I was infertile. Others said to me: "Wouldn't it be great for your research if you really *were* infertile?" Throughout the time of my field research, I was a married woman with no children in my late twenties. People I met in connection with my research almost always interrogated me about my own status and sometimes chastened me for daring to put off childbearing in the pursuit of a doctoral degree. In particular, women being treated in infertility clinics sometimes asked me whether I myself was also getting treatment in the clinic, since I did not have children and seemed to hang around there a lot. On many occasions, women chided me, saying, "Hurry up and have children! You don't want to end up in here with us!"

Deepak, my partner, belongs to a Kshatriya (Hindu warrior caste) family from Uttar Pradesh and grew up in Lucknow as part of a family with agricultural roots and a generation of mid-level government workers, educated but mostly not intellectual. We met during my first lengthy stay in Lucknow during a Fulbright research scholarship and married a couple of years later. At some point late in my initial doctoral research period and about five years into our marriage, after so many conversations about infertility, pregnancy loss, and infant and child death in women's lives, I remember walking down the road toward our home and thinking about our own prospects for children, which had never been a major focus of our attention up to that point in marriage. I grew up with few financial resources, but surrounded by extended family in rural western Pennsylvania, so agricultural metaphors about fertility, hesitation toward medical institutions, and emphasis on kin that I heard in Lucknow had resonated with me. That day, walking in the hot sun and dust, I remember feeling utterly convinced that, should we ever attempt to achieve conception, we would surely encounter some kind of problem. I thought my friends' joke would come true, even if it happened after I had concluded my field research.

The effect of many months spent talking with women in Lucknow about the uncertainties of biological reproduction and possible alternatives and the precarity of reproduction over the long haul—along with years spent reading about similar research in other places—had clearly taken a toll. After returning to the United States, the full-term and uncomplicated birth of our child in 2009 did alleviate some of these worries, but it also raised other questions for me about women's experiences in giving birth to and raising children. Accordingly, autoethnographic reflections on my life with my in-laws and their perspectives on "waiting for aulad" are part of the story in this account. I also focus attention on the legitimate concerns that women living in poverty in Lucknow have about when they can feel reasonably comfortable that they have been successful in creating *aulad*, even when they have not gone through any particular problems in conception, pregnancy, or birth.

The social locations I have occupied in Lucknow undoubtedly shaped the ways that people interacted with me. My position as a foreign researcher with an interest in Indo-Muslim culture and Urdu language, presumed by most to be of Christian origin, and a daughter-in-law in a high-caste Hindu family presented some challenges to my research but also helped to provide context for thinking about the larger picture of reproduction and social and religious life in contemporary India. My in-laws were impressed with my efforts to learn Urdu, a language that both of my partner's grandfathers knew well, but that no one in the current generations could read or write. At the same time, they were somewhat disturbed by my intentions to meet Muslim people across the social spectrum in Lucknow. These worries were partly associated with difference in class and religion but also with the movement of a female member of the household without anyone to accompany her as chaperone or guardian. I was fortunate that, without extreme protest on my part, they granted me a level of freedom of movement and freedom from regular household chores of which most Kshatriya daughters-in-law (*bahus*, bahū) of their class would have been jealous, although they sometimes expressed concern for my safety and insisted that I carry a mobile telephone.

The long-term entwinements of friends and kin I have experienced in Lucknow mean that I have always been immersed in local communities, and most intimately with the relatives, friends, and colleagues of my partner's family. Since my first trip, I have spent over four years living, studying, and conducting research in India. When I first met Deepak, I was spending nine months living with five hundred Indian students in a dorm for women studying at Lucknow University, where residents referred to each other as sisters—for elder sisters, Holly *didi*, Puja *didi*, and so on,

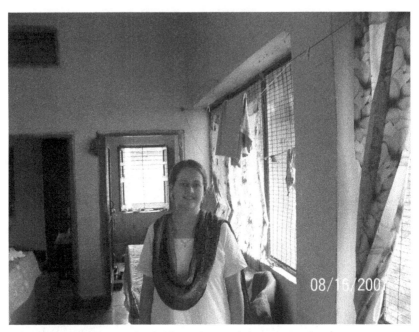

Figure b.3. At home in the field, Lucknow. (Photo by author.)

and given names for those younger—while I studied echoes of eighteenth- and nineteenth-century local history in contemporary Lucknow. Several of these women attended our wedding and took on roles that would otherwise be played by members of my natal family. In 2006–07, I lived in a multigenerational joint family transitioning from one home to another in Lucknow, which meant that the family was sometimes dispersed between two locations but always together to make important decisions.

Although I had a good measure of freedom, there were certain expectations the family wanted me to abide by to protect their, and my, honor (*izzat*, izzat). I had to fulfill, at least to some extent, the roles of a daughter-in-law (*bahu*), sister-in-law (*bhabhi*, bhābhī, elder brother's wife), aunt (*mami*, māmī, mother's brother's wife), and so on. Surveillance of my own fertility status became part of household conversations, in the form of questions such as "When are you going to make your mother-in-law a grandmother (*dadi*, dādī)?" Luckily for me, throughout the early years of my marriage, my mother-in-law took it upon herself to dismiss questions about children by explaining that I was still in school. These expectations would have been quite different, but not absent, had I been a foreign son-in-law, or *damad* (dāmād).

Sometimes my research benefited from my being part of frank conversations about fertility and everyday life, including household disputes and intimate details about fertility management. At other times, I could be ready to head off for a meeting somewhere when relatives, associates, or old friends of the family would turn up and need to be received with chai (tea) and conversation. During my previous long stay, while living in the women's hostel at Lucknow University, I also experienced many such moments and numerous thwarted exits from our shared living space. In the long run, some of my most valuable insights came through taking those pauses to enjoy the company of and conversation with the young women with whom I lived. So, too, was my experience participating in the life of the household. I have been fortunate that the times of frustration and pain have, so far, tended to be balanced with moments of contentment and joy. Being surrounded by family has protected me from much of the danger and violence that researchers out of place, and especially women, face all too often during fieldwork. The richness of these interactions has also helped to moderate the intense loneliness that many anthropologists report during extended periods of fieldwork, and it has reminded me to keep the vibrance of living and doing kinship, including emotional aspects of relatedness, in view.

These dynamics have changed over the course of my marriage and the unfolding of life events. The challenges and limitations of being part of a local family also suited my research, since there was no colony of infertile people for me to join as a round-the-clock participant-observer. I could not simply transplant myself in any neighborhood twenty-four hours a day to study it holistically. This movement, however, also meant that I could compare and contrast my experiences with those of the women I met in Lucknow who were negotiating their own family situations, while being careful not to assume that my perspectives could easily translate into theirs (akin to the perspective sensitively portrayed by Robert Desjarlais [1992,14–30] while explaining his work with shamans in Nepal). My history of intimacies in Lucknow has been a boon to my research and to my life. It inspired me to work even harder to gain the fluency in Hindi/ Urdu that would be crucial to my ability to live in my household day-to-day and to do my research without having a translator present. The presence of a translator could very well have made difficult conversations about reproduction impossible. I made a point of learning to read and write both Hindi and Urdu, and to hone the pronunciation and rhythm of my speech.

In 2010, I returned for another extended stay in Lucknow in yet another new position—still a wife and daughter-in-law, but now also the mother of a young child. I dealt with the challenges of balancing writing far away from campus resources with somewhat erratic access to electricity and internet facilities. On the other hand, I was able to share childcare duties and running the household with several enthusiastic family members. I could discuss the framing of my writing with family members, friends, and other interlocutors. Since then, I have returned to Lucknow as often as possible with my partner and my growing child. These sustained—and sustaining—continuing entwinements and interactions with people in Lucknow as I have grown into my profession and into parenting have contributed much to this ethnography.

NOTES

1. Quote from study participant in group conversation in Gehumandi basti, Lucknow, June 2007. In this chapter and throughout the book, quotations come from interviews conducted during fieldwork in India from 2005 to 2007 and 2015 to 2016. Other references draw on participant

observation and casual interactions across many stays in India from 1998 onward.

2. World Population Prospects 2019: Highlights, accessed June 3, 2021, https://population.un.org/wpp/Publications/Files/WPP2019_10 KeyFindings.pdf. While these figures are highly contingent, as of 2019, India was predicted to overtake China in population around 2027.

3. Partners in Health, organization cofounded by Paul Farmer, on Twitter, for one example of this popular internet meme: https://twitter .com/pih/status/224177665551237121.

4. The reproductive justice movement continues to expand and flourish in the United States. To learn more, see, for example: ACRJ 2005; Ross 2006; Ross and Solinger 2017; Ross et al. 2017; Davis 2019; Luna and Luker 2013; Scott 2021, and the online presence of organizations such as Sister-Song, Black Mamas Matter, and their partner organizations across the country.

5. https://www.sistersong.net/reproductive-justice accessed 09 June 2021.

6. Census India 2011: accessed August 17, 2015, http://www.census2011 .co.in/census/district/528-lucknow.html.

7. Census India 2011: accessed July 16, 2015, http://www.censusindia .gov.in/2011-prov-results/data_files/up/Census2011Data%20Sheet-UP.pdf. According to popular media, this relative trend continues as the population of Uttar Pradesh continues to grow. See, for example, Kopf and Varathan 2017.

8. BIMARU states, according to this shorthand: Bihar, Madhya Pradesh, Rajasthan, Uttar Pradesh. Demographer Ashish Bose is publicly credited with coining this term in the 1980s. "Ashish Bose, Who Coined Bimaru, Dies at 84," *Indian Express Online*, April 8, 2014.

9. Also see PBS Online *World in the Balance* website at http://www .pbs.org/wgbh/nova/worldbalance/.

10. Sample Registration System Statistical Report 2018: accessed May 27, 2021, https://censusindia.gov.in/vital_statistics/SRS_Reports_2018 .html, chap. 3, p. 78. Statewise comparison: Bihar, 3.2; Madhya Pradesh, 2.7; Rajasthan, 2.5; Kerala, 1.7; West Bengal, 1.5.

11. In comparative perspective: Afghanistan at 50/1,000, Pakistan at 62/1,000, Nepal at 34/1,000 (all of these rates have fallen rapidly in the last five years), contrasted with the United States at 5.7/1,000, Canada at 4.7/1,000, Cuba at 4.0/1,000, and Sweden at 1.8/1,000. *2020 World Population Data Sheet*, accessed May 29, 2021, https://interactives.prb.org/2020

-wpds/download-files/. However, there is considerable variation in the rates among regions and classes in India.

12. Sample Registration System Statistical Report 2018: accessed May 27, 2021, https://censusindia.gov.in/vital_statistics/SRS_Reports_2018 .html, chap. 4, p. 137.

13. Sample Registration System. Compendium of India's Fertility and Mortality Indicators ,1971–2013: accessed April 10, 2022, https://censusindia .gov.in/vital_statistics/Compendium/Srs_data.html.

14. Reports from Government of India Ministry of Health and Family Welfare on rates from 2010–2012: accessed August 18, 2015, http://pib.nic .in/newsite/PrintRelease.aspx?relid=103446 and on 2016–18, accessed June 4, 2021, https://www.pib.gov.in/PressReleasePage.aspx?PRID =1697441.

15. The film is based on a short story by the same name by Premchand, one of the most prominent early twentieth-century writers in Urdu and Hindi.

16. *Kaba* refers to the empty black structure around which Muslims circumambulate during the Hajj pilgrimage, and toward which they orient during daily prayers. Couplet cited in Awadhwasi Lala Sitaram, *Ayodhya ka Itihas*, Praya (1932) and quoted in Mohan 1997: 151.

17. See also Hasan and Menon (2004) and Engineer (1995).

18. For example, India: Jeffery and Jeffery 2006; Ram 2001. China: Greenhalgh 2010, 2008; Greenhalgh and Winckler 2005. Italy: Krause and Marchesi 2007; Krause 2005. Europe: Douglass 2005. Greece: Paxson 2004. Israel: Kanaaneh 2002; Kahn 2000. Romania: Kligman 1998. Singapore: Heng and Devan 1992. Global: Hartmann 1987.

19. Sadiq, Kalbe. Lecture at Shah Najaf Imambara, Lucknow, 2006. The "quality over quantity" expression has also been a common one in global demographic and family-planning literature.

20. See also Weigl 2010.

21. Refers to the geographical area between the Yamuna River in northern India near Delhi and the Ganga (Ganges) River, which runs through north-central India, including Uttar Pradesh.

ONE

AULAD

Reproductive Desires

LABORED RELATIONS

Qudsia Baji

Qudsia baji (bājī) is an elderly woman I met in 2007 when I attended meetings of a ladies' organization in Lucknow, whose membership, although open to all women, largely consisted of Muslim women.[1] From their dress and bearing at the meetings, these women seemed to come from a variety of class backgrounds and, judging by their dress, to observe varying degrees of purdah. The most observant hid their faces from photographers covering the events for local media, while others openly entered the meeting—which was limited to women, media staff, and the men who ran the sound system—without any special head covering. Most women, however, wore *saris* (sāṛī), *shalwar kameez* (shalvār kamīz, a tunic with loose pants), or, very occasionally, *churidaar kameez* (churidar kamīz, a tunic with tight pants), not Western dress.

A close associate and employee of the head of the organization, Qudsia baji immediately volunteered to talk with me about her experiences of dealing with childlessness. Her story began with her marriage nearly forty years earlier. She did not dwell on medical treatment or strategies, either ritual or therapeutic, to alleviate her childlessness. Her main focus in recalling her experiences was on the relationships within her marital home and how her in-laws treated her.

After two years of marriage without giving birth, people in her *sasural* (sasurāl), her husband's side of the family, started to talk. She said that she was married for twelve years without giving birth. Then she became pregnant and gave birth to a baby that she believed to be stillborn but later found out had lived for several minutes after being born. Qudsia baji was only around fourteen when her marriage was arranged with a man at least twenty years her senior, so even after twelve years of marriage, she would have only been in her mid-to-late-twenties. After that, she said, although she was fond of children (*bacchon ka shauq tha*), another six years passed before she gave birth to a son, who lived (in 2007, he was about twenty-one). Amid these reproductive travails, she tried at least a couple of times, unsuccessfully, to adopt a child from within her extended family.

The head of the ladies' organization, Shabana baji, knew Qudsia baji well. Shabana baji cast doubts on Qudsia baji's version of her reproductive history, saying that she doubted whether Qudsia baji's son was actually her own because he did not show any attachment toward his parents. I note this not to suggest that either of them was not telling the truth but to emphasize the understandings of family relationships indicated by Shabana baji's comments. Her evaluation implies not that he was a *bad* son, because he failed to perform his appropriate role as a dutiful and caring son, but that he must not be their *real* son at all. Her comment also underscores the legitimate reasons why people suffering from infertility in this cultural context hide their treatment strategies and eventual outcomes from others, particularly if they eventually get children through biomedical infertility treatments, especially assisted reproductive technologies that involve donor gametes or surrogacy; or if they adopt a child.

In our conversations, Qudsia baji presented herself as a person
who worked hard to maintain herself and to help others, even
though they often forgot her when she needed help. She focused
on the difficulties she encountered after marriage and before children through problems with her in-laws, especially her mother-
in-law (*saas*, sās), her husband's sister (*nand*, nand), and her husband's younger brother's wife (*devrani*, devrānī). Although she
criticized her husband for his behavior with his family and his
failure, from her perspective, to vocally take issue with the treatment she received from others, she emphasized that he did not
push her or abuse her because of their childless state. Instead, he
offered her comfort in private. She explained,

> He [husband] never said, "We don't have any children" or, "I'll
> leave you." . . . One day my mother-in-law took him aside and said
> to him, "Leave her . . . I'll get you married again. . . ." His habit is
> such that he never says anything to anyone, even now he doesn't
> say anything against his elders . . . he only argues with me . . .
> he couldn't even say to his mother, "What are you saying?" So I
> began to get worried. Then he said, "Why are you getting so wor-
> ried? There's nothing like that, that I will leave you or get married
> a second time. Let her say what she wants . . . there are children
> in the family. . . ." I never had any complaints about him, but I did
> from every other direction. . . . My methods, my manners, my get-
> ting up and sitting down . . . in everything, objections were raised
> against me, but he never said anything. (Interview July 23, 2007)

Even though she criticized her husband for his silence, Qudsia
baji emphasized that she, too, remained silent, tolerating slights
and criticisms from her husband's relatives. She did remember
one incident that drew attention to her childless state in a way
that hurt her more than the daily nitpicking that seems to have
been the main feature of her interactions with her in-laws. It happened at the husband's elder brother's daughter's wedding (*jeth*,
jeth: husband's elder brother; *jeth ki larki*, jeth kī laṛkī: his daughter). She worked hard to help prepare for the wedding, sewing,

cooking, and organizing the house. She explained that she took a major role in getting everything ready for the wedding, and no one was concerned that her participation would have any negative impact on the girl who was to be married.

> I didn't confront anything, I endured it.... What can I call myself.... I bore it myself.... The clothes worn at the time of the *nikah* [Muslim marriage ceremony] are considered to be the most important.... I sewed all of her clothes, all of that girl's clothes... at that time, I wasn't a barren woman [*banjh*] ... putting away, picking up all of the food and supplies.... My husband's elder brother was my father's friend, so he considered me to be like his daughter, and he called me by my name. So, if he asked for something even at midnight, I accepted it, and did everything. (Interview July 23, 2007)

At the time of the marriage ceremony, when the bride was being dressed and prepared with special bridal jewelry, Qudsia baji's husband's elder brother's wife (her *jethani*, jethānī) singled her out and asked her not to help the bride wear the large circular nose ring (*nath*) that is a customary part of bridal attire in Uttar Pradesh among both Hindus and Muslims. Her *jethani* also said that the bride should not enter into the kind of married state that Qudsia baji had. After all the work she had done to prepare the household for the event, and even though many years had passed since the incident, Qudsia baji still felt bitter about her *jethani's* words, saying,

> But at the time of the *nikah* I became a barren woman [*banjh*]. So, the girl didn't wear any silver jewelry placed by my hand... so I got up and left that place. Then the whole matter got spread around the household. Shaqib's wife has gone ... now Shaqib's wife has gone, so all to work has come to a standstill.... He [husband] called from downstairs, "Qudsia, Qudsia, come down ... I'm telling you, come downstairs." I came down on the sly, silently, and I started crying. I said, "I've put up with so much poverty, but today, why did she bring up my happily married state [*suhag*]? If she had mentioned the matter of our children [*aulad*],

then it wouldn't have mattered." Fine, I'm this sort of person, so just let me be like this. (Interview July 23, 2007)

Qudsia baji seems to have taken on the burden of blame for their childless state, along with a substantial amount of the household labor. Even though she had carved out a space for herself in the everyday operation of the household, being snubbed on such a joyous occasion both stung her pride and highlighted the complex and delicate nature of relationships within the *sasural*, particularly among the women living there together. In infertility clinics in Lucknow, younger women also shared many stories about managing their social and familial relationships as women who had not yet fulfilled the reproductive ideals embraced by themselves, their families, or society as they saw it. The complexities of navigating family relationships, reproductive ideals, and reproductive desires were not a relic of the past.

The stories, songs, and popular literature from women in Lucknow discussed in this chapter show the particular shapes that reproductive desires take in North India. Context makes all the difference for understanding reproductive desires, otherwise identified by demographers as fertility intentions. In North India, reproductive desires include specific ideals of the relationship between children and the families who raise them, which the term *aulad* expresses most fully. Understanding family-making and the implications of infertility and childlessness that make hiding unconventional reproductive efforts attractive in North India requires expanding the frame of analysis beyond women of childbearing age and beyond married couples. The reasons for taking a broader view are not because childbearing frequently happens outside of marriage—nonmarital fertility is highly stigmatized—but because the networks of family members involved in generating and fulfilling child desire are much wider, and their opinions and actions strongly influence people wishing for children. This chapter, then, is a meditation on agency in child desire—whose desire?—and on the contours of desire—which children are desirable? At an even more fundamental level, it is an examination of kinship—how people understand, make, and remake bonds of relatedness in the face of reproductive disruption (Inhorn 2007).

Based on the prayers and blessings of a father, the song *"Baabul ki Duaen"* (Daddy's Prayers, babul kī duāen) has been a standard soundtrack for North Indian weddings for decades. Like most popular tunes in North India, it was composed for and made famous by a film, in this case, the 1968 Bollywood film *Neel Kamal* (Blue Lotus) (Maheshwary et al. [1968] 1999). With lyrics by Urdu poet Sahir Ludhianvi performed with appropriately overwrought emotion by Mohammad Rafi, the song is meant to exemplify both the despair and the hope of a loving father sending his daughter on her way to her *sasural*, the home of her in-laws.

> Go with your Daddy's prayers, go, may you receive a world of happiness
> May you get so much love in your in-laws' place [*sasural*] that you never think of your own parents' home [*maike*]
> Daddy's prayers . . .
> *Baabul ki duaaen leti ja, ja tujh ko sukhi sansaar mile*
> *Maike ki kabhi na yaad aae, sasuraal men itana pyaar mile*
> *Baabul ki duaaen . . .* (Maheshwary et al. [1968] 1999)[2]

The song's lyrics and emotional rendering focus on the time of *vidai/rukhsati*, the conclusion of the marriage rituals, when new brides formally leave for their marital homes with a great show of sobbing from their natal families. The unique plaintive tone of the *shehnai*, a distinctive woodwind instrument with a shape resembling an oboe or clarinet, the slow tempo, and the singer's voice evoke emotional responses. So do lyrics that bespeak a father's longing, wishes, and doubt about whether the prayers and blessings he offers will be fulfilled, even though it is usually a

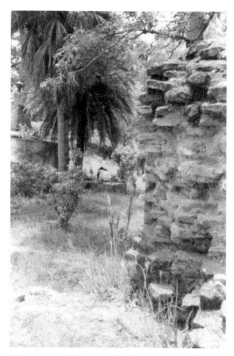

Figure 1.1. Historical sites such as the ruins of the nineteenth-century British Residency offer opportunities for tourism and for intimacy. (Photo by author.)

bride's female relatives who weep most openly and copiously at her departure.

The vast majority of marriages, particularly in the North Indian system, are still arranged by the close relatives of the prospective bride and groom and marriage remains one of the most significant concerns of parents for their daughters. Many parents of daughters consider finding a "suitable boy" (after Vikram Seth's 1993 novel)—and beyond that, a suitable family—for their daughters as their greatest duty in their daughters' lives, eclipsing the fulfillment of educational or professional aspirations. Framing the reproductive aspirations, desires, and decisions of married couples in North India within the context of the extended family shows how these relationships influence the experiences of women in their reproductive lives. In this chapter, I focus on cases in which childbirth does not follow soon after marriage to emphasize the interplay of various house-hold members and the ways procreation can be a major factor in the distribution of power within the household. Although these contests for power and control take place mainly among women, their implications reverberate among all members of the household.

The plotlines of many Indian films and television shows (seri-als) revolve around relationships within households and in par-ticular around the role of the daughter-in-law (*bahu*) in her mari-tal household. New daughters-in-law are often seen as threats to family unity. As outsiders, they should be slowly integrated into their marital households, with great care given to making sure the son's loyalty remains with his natal family, rather than with his wife. Conveying awareness of the precarious position of his daughter, the father in "*Baabul ki Duaen*" still sends her off but with his fervent wishes for her well-being:

> May the moments of your life pass in the pleasant cool shade
> May no thorn ever be able to prick your feet, my darling girl
> May sorrows stay far away from that doorway too, to which your path leads
> Daddy's prayers . . .
> *Beeten tere jeevan ki ghadiyaan, Aaraam ki thandi chhaanvon men*
> *Kaanta bhi na chubhane paae kabhi, Meri laadali tere paanvon men*
> *Us dvaar se bhi dukh dur rahen, Jis dvaar se tera dvaar mile*
> *Baabul ki duaaen . . .* (Maheshwary et al. [1968] 1999)[3]

As in many parts of the world where patrilineal, patrilocal systems of kinship and marriage predominate, social-science research in North India shows that women often enter their marital households, and especially joint, multigenerational fam-ilies, as low-status members of the household (Das Gupta 1995;

Jeffery et al. 1989). In-laws tend to regard new daughters-in-law, at least initially, with some measure of suspicion. Daughters-in-law are expected to prove their loyalty to their marital households through labor, deferential service to other members of the household, and childbirth. Indian psychoanalyst Sudhir Kakar (1978) described a stereotypical ideal of the new daughter-in-law in her marital home, highlighting reasons why the father in the song *"Baabul ki Duaen"* might feel doubt and anxiety about the impending departure of his daughter on the path to her *sasural* (in-laws' place):

> Unflinchingly and without complaint, the new daughter-in-law is required to perform some of the heaviest household chores, which may mean getting up well before dawn and working till late at night. Any mistakes or omissions on her part are liable to incur sarcastic references to her abilities, her looks or her upbringing in her mother's home. For it must be noted once again that the new bride constitutes a very real threat to the unity of the extended family. . . . The nature of the "danger" she personi-fies can perhaps best be suggested by such questions as: Will the young wife cause her husband to neglect his duties as a son? As a brother? A nephew? An uncle? Will social tradition and family pressure be sufficient to keep the husband-wife bond from devel-oping to a point where it threatens the interests of other family members? (Kakar 1978, 74)

Even though these representations of extended family rela-tions are decades old, the song continues to circulate in popular culture, and its themes continue to resonate for many people liv-ing in North India in the realms of fears, ideals, and, sometimes, experience. Kakar's analysis draws heavily on Hindu mythology, as well as on his own understandings of Indian culture, and fo-cuses mainly on Hindu ideology, with little space devoted to the differences that emerge across religious backgrounds. Portrayals of daughters-in-law in popular culture rarely differentiate these experiences by religious background, and, indeed, many of the role expectations within joint families bear striking commonalities. According to accounts of the lives of women in their marital homes in anthropological and demographic literature on South Asia, giving birth to children, and especially sons, increases the status of daughters-in-law, until they, in turn, become mothers-in-law who can influence the behavior of their own daughters-in-law (Das Gupta 1995; Patel 1994; Bumiller 1990). From Tamil Nadu, South India, Margaret Trawick offers another perspective that could serve as a model both for new brides and for children brought into families in less conventional ways, focusing on how "adjustment" (*pallikam*) happens in that part of the country (Trawick 1990). There are, indeed, other models for forging bonds that have some relevance, through other ways of defining kinship ties and the sharing of substances like breast milk, water, food, residence, and care, as well as friendship, but within cultural and legal limits.

In the shifting realities of contemporary South Asia, the increased migration of young men and women for job opportunities, changing norms of gender relations, spousal relationships, and women's growing employment outside the home challenge ideals about family relationships (Lamb 2000; Brunson 2016). However, the model of deference still holds strong ideological power, especially among members of the older generations. Older women may, indeed, be caught between ideas about women's advancement and equality that would encourage them to expect less from their daughters-in-law and memories of dealing with their own in-laws' old-age care with the comfort of thoughts that one day they would receive care from their own daughters-in-law. The failure of such care to materialize can sting, and compromises in the form of care from hired servants can fail to deliver anticipated physical and emotional support.

WOMEN'S HONOR, FAMILY HONOR,
AND THE *SASURAL*

Women's behavior in their natal and marital households serves as a particularly potent barometer by which other family members and society (*samaj*) judge family honor (*izzat*, see also Mandelbaum 1988). Many of my interlocutors in Lucknow commonly referred to *samaj* to talk about normative expectations, in accordance with or against personal beliefs based on their own experiences and social position. Their status as daughters-in-law in their marital households and the respect garnered by entire households depend not only on the fecundity of daughters-in-law but also on their conduct with family members and household visitors. Surveillance of the everyday activities of daughters and daughters-in-law, both by family members and others with whom women regularly come into contact in their neighborhoods, schools, and/or places of work, is extremely high. This is most true in comparison with the surveillance of men's activities in general, and particularly in regions, castes, and religious groups with a strong history of the practice of purdah. *Purdah* literally means *curtain*, but it also refers to the separation of the sexes by secluding women. There are several varieties of purdah practices in North India historically and at present that range from the seclusion of women in a separate living area in a home (*mardana* and *zenana*, men's and women's quarters); to limiting the movement of women outside the home, with variation depending on a woman's age, marital status, and presence in her natal home or in-laws home; to requiring particular modes of dress and covering the body, particularly the head, in the presence of particular family members or nonfamily members; to recommending certain standards of dress, movement, and conduct for women (Vatuk 1982; Papanek and Minault 1982).

Even in communities without formal purdah practices in North India, it is still common for women, especially young women, to be held to a different standard than men in terms of where they go, whom they meet, and the activities in which they partake. For example, there are widespread significant differences in the level of social criticism generated by the consumption of alcohol, smoking, and sexual activity, depending on the sex of the person involved. Men may be criticized, but are easily excused for such acts. But for most women, these activities, and situations that are likely to lead to speculation about their engaging in such activities, are either strictly avoided or conducted with a strong view toward maintaining secrecy. The possible consequences vary for women, but when looking at people of similar social status, they tend to be more significant for women than for men.

When I lived in a hostel (dormitory) for women studying at Lucknow University for nine months while conducting research just after I graduated from college, in 2000–2001, I learned this lesson in short order. About five hundred women lived in the hostel. Even though they lived away from home and could move freely around the university and the city, hostel regulations limited women's movements. Women lived under a daily curfew stipulating that they return home by 8:00 p.m. and sign a register kept outside the entryway to the dining hall. With permission obtained by getting a special letter of application approved by the hostel "warden," a professor as known for her outspoken nature and commanding presence as for her elaborate saris and bindis (dots placed on the forehead between the eyebrows), women could stay out until 9:30 p.m. After that, the hostel gates were locked, and women had to plead with the night watchmen to let them in, since a thick concrete wall topped with barbed wire enclosed the entire hostel campus and its several dormitory buildings. At 10:00 p.m., the doors to each dormitory inside the hostel were locked until morning, preventing anyone from entering or exiting the building overnight. Students always hurried to fill their water bottles from the hand pump or tube wells in the campus courtyards before they were locked in for the night. Women could be fined 25 rupees (then about 60 cents, enough money to buy a cheap meal) for failing to sign in, and their relatives might be notified about their absence. Male visitors could enter public outdoor areas of the hostel only during set visiting hours, and they could never go inside the residential areas.

Most people I knew in the hostel thought these rules to be sensible and necessary, even though there were no such regulations for the men's dormitories on the other end of the university campus. The warden explained that parents had entrusted their daughters' care to the hostel staff, so they were obligated to care for the students, "inmates" of the hostel, as honorary daughters. Despite all these provisions, I still heard people talk disparagingly about women who lived in the hostel. The freedom of movement and freedom from the constant supervision of relatives indexed by residence in the hostel became indicators of their less-than-ideal moral character, regardless of their actions as individuals. Hostel girls had a reputation that preceded them. While I can't argue that all the residents were completely innocent in their personal conduct, or that none of them participated in relationships, such details proved largely incidental in a place where purdah still had strong ideological power.

In Uttar Pradesh, women's residence after marriage is most commonly patrilocal. Newly married women live with their husbands in her *sasural*, the family home focused on the most senior man, or in a separate home near their husband's workplace, especially if this is far from the *sasural*. Whether women work after marriage or not depends on their family's class status, and whether or not a bride will be permitted or compelled to hold a job after marriage may be a point of negotiation in arranged marriages. Among Hindus, new brides are usually strangers to their in-laws, although in arranged marriages, they generally belong to the same caste group, with more or less strict adherence to regulations about the allowable degree of relationship permissible, sub-caste (*jati*) affiliation, and village and patrilineal clan (*gotra*) exogamy (marrying outside, Karve 1994 [1953], 51–63) that aim to enforce distance. Among Muslims, marriages among strangers can and do happen, especially through newspaper advertisements and online resources such as the matchmaking website Shaadi.com (which translates as wedding.com). However, marriage within kin groups, such as cousin marriage at various degrees, also occurs frequently (Ahmad 1978, 193; Husain 1976, 68; Ahmad 1976). According to Islamic and Indian law, Muslim men have the option of unilaterally divorcing any wife or of marrying up to four women without divorcing the previous wife/ wives. Polygyny is now uncommon but not unheard of among Hindus or Muslims in India (Iyer 2002), yet it is legally available only for Muslim men. Polyandry, a practice whereby one woman has multiple husbands at one time, is not an option for Muslim women, and women's rights to divorce are limited, as well as socially stigmatized (see Vatuk 2003 on *khula'* divorce). Complexities of marital law mean that polygyny is not legal for Hindus in India and divorce is comparatively more difficult to obtain.

In North Indian family interactions that I have observed over two decades, discussion about the intrigue of relationships between various family members, gifts given and received (or not), forms of address, greetings given or withheld, and the quality of food and drink produced by daughters-in-law compose an enormous part of household conversations. Although such discussions may also include the activities of friends and neighbors, the most intense attention focuses on members of one's own extended family. In general, discussions about family relations occupy a much more prominent place in household conversations than would be the case in most American families. In part, these conversations ascertain the appropriate level of reciprocity for future interactions with family and friends, within general conventions, based on marriage, seniority, level of government post, and so on, which designate some people as givers and others as takers. In the case of family relations, much of the Lévi-Straussian anthropological framework of wife-givers and wife-takers applies to the distribution of gifts and respect, although others have questioned this (Raheja 1988; Vatuk 1975).[4] For example, how many kilograms of sweets were given? What kind? Were the rotis (round flatbread) round enough; were they thin or thick; were they partly raw, burned, or perfectly cooked? Whose feet were touched, and who merely received a greeting, with folded hands, of "namaste"? Was the health of other household members asked after? These mundane tasks and selections demonstrate the level of respect accorded to particular friends and/or relatives, and injured parties may remember perceived slights for years. Family members remember, in incredibly detailed ways, the gifts given and received at previous social functions, such as relatives' wed- dings, and these exchanges form an important basis of this kin work (di Leonardo 1987), particularly on the part of women in the household. Beyond reciprocity, these details form part of an in- tricate calculus of the distribution of respect (*izzat*) among fam- ily members and friends. Good conduct, or refinement (*tehzeeb, tameez*), displayed by family members can also help to increase family *izzat* (respect or honor), while bad conduct (*badtameezi*) can harm a family's reputation, and especially that of the particu- lar family members involved.

A sizeable social-science literature, much of it carried out through national and international population agencies deter- mined to shrink the average number of births per woman in In- dia, has examined the effects of the patrilocal system of residence on the health of young married women and their children, as well as on women's ideals and actual practices regarding family size, birth control (notable among them Jeffery et al. 1989; Srini- vas and Ramaswamy 1977), and food intake during pregnancy (Vallianatos 2006; Das Gupta 1995; Nag 1994). In studies with a strong quantitative orientation, cases of infertility rarely garner much attention, since, in large-scale studies, infertility levels and comparative prevalence of infertility across India rarely figure as statistically significant factors (Jejeebhoy 1998, 17, 23). Even when ethnographic interviews, participant observation, and other ethnographic methods are the main methodological tools used in research on birth and population, infertility problems and beliefs about them have rarely been given focused attention as an important factor in considering men's and women's opinions about the age at marriage, ideal family size, and appropriate methods of birth control, if any. This has been a significant gap in research over the last several decades, even though any case of infertility becomes magnified in importance for families experiencing it personally.

Such studies, however, show the need to look beyond the married couple for the locus of decision-making authority in matters of reproduction, and especially point to the important roles that mothers-in-law play in influencing the fertility of their sons and daughters-in-law. This can include close surveillance of menstrual cycles (*taarikh* or *mahina*, words meaning date or month), of eating and bathing habits, and of other routine aspects of everyday life. Studies examining the cultural dynamics of contraception, for example, point out that women feel the need to hide their birth control pills and their daily consumption of them from their mothers-in-law, in case they seize the pills or subject them to heavy criticism for taking them (Char et al. 2010; International Institute for Population Sciences 2001).

If the birth of children is a primary way for daughters-in-law to increase their status in their marital homes, especially if they are not working for pay and/or do not bring substantial wealth from their natal homes, then the absence of living children can be a significant threat to their security within their marital households. According to Kakar, "Numerous passages in legends and epics vividly describe the sufferings of the souls of departed ancestors if a couple remain childless and thus unable to guarantee the performance of the rituals prescribed for salvation. . . . Subjectively, in the world of feminine psychological experience, pregnancy is a deliverance from the insecurity, doubt and shame of infertility: 'Better be mud than a barren woman', goes one proverb" (Kakar 1978, 77).

Kakar moves effortlessly from discussing a childless couple to a barren woman, without mentioning the possibility that the infertility could be due to male-factor infertility. The stigma of infertility in South Asia falls first and most heavily on the woman (Grey 2017). However, if a childless man opts for divorce and/or remarriage, his fertility status might be questioned if the new wife also fails to produce children. Kakar highlights the tentative nature of marriage bonds, not only between husband and wife but also between wife and members of the husband's extended family. Family members expect the birth of children to fortify these bonds, particularly by adding sons to the family.

In Lucknow, many women suffering from infertility defended their husbands and suggested that sharing the experience of seeking children strengthened their marital bond, regardless of the cause of their infertility, even though in some cases this intimacy came at the cost of close relationships with other members of the extended family. In Egypt, Inhorn reported increased levels of intimacy between husbands and wives seeking infertility treatment (Inhorn 2006, 1996). She documented other cases in which husbands faced with the prospects of continuing to live in a childless marriage opted to divorce the first wife and marry a younger woman who agreed to go through extensive infertility treatment—often intracytoplasmic sperm injection—with them (Inhorn 2003, especially chap. 8). When husbands and wives travel on their "quests for children" without their extended families, the experience of infertility provides a rather unique opportunity for husbands and wives to share time and secrets, away from the eyes of other household members and out of earshot of their criticisms.

THE SASURAL IS A MARIGOLD

"*Genda Phool*," an A. R. Rahman song from the 2009 film *Delhi-6* (*Dilli-Chhe*), directed by Rakeysh Omprakash Mehra and starring Waheeda Rehman, Abhishek Bachchan, and Sonam Kapoor, presents the *sasural* in another way, distinct from the world of "Daddy's Prayers" ("*Babul ki Duaen*"). The song, performed as cast members dance on the rooftop of a home in densely populated, crumbling Old Delhi, focuses on women's lives after marriage. In light, village-inflected, sparse language, it examines the relationships among family members in the *sasural* from a daughter-in-law's perspective. The lyrics summarize complications new brides navigate in their marital homes, the teasing and taunts that can be accompanied by unexpected criticism and solidarity (Mehra et al. 2009).[5]

"*Genda Phool*" reflects changes in aesthetics in film and music in recent decades. Songs like "*Baabul ki Duaen*" continue to circulate, but they stand alongside songs that portray marriage in a lighter, less serious manner. In "*Genda Phool*," the lyrics of complaint and enjoyment are set to a dance beat that fits in well on popular television programs and in urban clubs, and the characters are singing and joking about the *sasural* with a woman who is yet unmarried. In the song, the bride has left behind her father's courtyard—*baabul ka angana*—and has entered the tangled entwinements of relationships in her husband's family's home.

The lyrics in Hindi film songs can be difficult to understand, sometimes because they draw from a heavily Urdu-register vocabulary of words that are not often used conversationally, and sometimes because the quality of lyrics is sacrificed to a good beat, which showcases the dance performance of an "item girl" who has a small role in the film, or ignores the importance of the film's music. This song, if not the movie, was a hit in India. Even a glance at the YouTube commenters, generally Hindi/Urdu speakers around the world, makes clear their confusion over the meanings of the phrase "*sasural genda phool*." For example,

Cutiepari (United States, likes *Twilight*) said: @warrio619: sasural means husband's house and genda phool is a type of flower which is commonly used in wedding garlands

Imrangogi (no information) said: @warrio619
the arrangement of petals of flower is called inflorescence . . . here in this song it means my family is like flower (genda phool . . . a complex arranged flower). there are lot of difficulties in this world but she says that she is facing the difficulties wd courage as her family support her . . . she is living for her love.[6]

107Rainbow (a teenager from Kerala, south India) said: Genda Phool (Marigolds) are complex flowers because its actually inflorescent in nature, which, by definition, is a complicated arrangement of flowers on a branch. So in the song, the girl compares her Sasural to this flower, because of all the complex relationship she shares with her mother-in-law, brother-in-law and sister-in-law. In spite of all the troubles, she loves being there for the love of her husband.[7]

The online users offering their interpretations of *"sasural genda phool"* come from different backgrounds and parts of the world. A common element running through the comments, which also aligns with the song's other lyrics, is the idea that daughters-in-law stand in a number of different relationships, which take stereotypical forms. Bright orange—nearly saffron—marigolds are ubiquitous in North Indian Hindu marriage ceremonies to decorate marriage halls and *mandaps* (tent) beneath which the main marriage rituals take place. The flowers are strung together to make garlands for the bride and groom and used in *puja* worship offerings. The entwinement of the flower's petals, their imbrications into one complete flower reflect the many dimensions of relationships young women might encounter in their *sasural*. Family members, for example, always interested in what would otherwise be personal business, resemble the close formation of the marigold. Here, the multiplicity of meanings gives a sense of the complexity belied by the simple language used. The confusion shows how particular listeners might differ in their interpretations based on their familiarity with the language and its regional

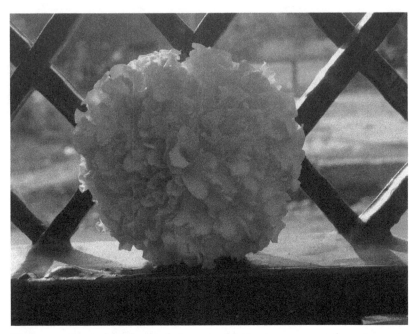

Figure 1.2. *Sasural genda phool*: A marigold sits atop a gate at the entrance to the family home, Lucknow, India. (Photo by author.)

variations and their understandings of what women experience after marriage. The tangled web of relationships in marital homes informs many Hindi films and television shows. After the release of *Delhi-6*, the cable network Star Plus launched a Hindi-language serial, similar to a soap opera or telenovela, called "*Sasural Genda Phool*," which aired from 2010 to 2012. The show's website lists 573 episodes available for online viewing.[8]

When a marriage takes place, the family fertility clock begins to tick. Family members wait for announcements and search for signs of impending family expansion. In the close quarters in which most joint families live, attempts by daughters-in-law to conceal changes in mood, appetite, appearance, and other initial signs of pregnancy, including the abandonment of menstruation management, create doubt, especially among women in the family. As time goes by without announcements, family members, friends, acquaintances, and even strangers begin to speculate and ask questions. Any good news (*khush khabri*)? When are you going to give us good news? When are you going to make me an auntie (or uncle)? How long since the marriage took place? Newly married couples cannot live with the illusion that no one is keeping tabs on their fertility status, especially if good news is not soon forthcoming.

The idea of voluntarily waiting for an extended time after marriage before pursuing parenthood is still uncommon in India, although it is becoming more prevalent as larger numbers of women pursue advanced educational degrees and professional aspirations. The age at marriage has risen, which delays childbearing, but most families still assume that children will result soon after marriage, regardless of the new couple's aspirations. Educational and career considerations are more often reasons for delaying marriage than for delaying fertility after marriage. As in many areas of life (Snell-Rood 2015), on the topics of both marriage and childbearing, women in Lucknow repeated that "X won't let you live." In other words, X, which could represent family, neighbors, or society in general, would not let women live without marrying, and, once married, they would not let women live without having children. Defying these conventions could lead to nagging, criticism, and gossip about women, their "character," and possibly their family background. Taking a different path would require the courage and ability to disregard commentary from others.

THE MEANINGS OF *AULAD*

औलाद

aulad [A.: pl. of *valad*], f. children; offspring; descendants (McGregor [1993] 1997, 150)

When I first started this project, I understood the term *aulad*
to be roughly equivalent to the word *baccha* (baccā; feminine
form *bacchi*), which in Hindi/Urdu means "child" but in everyday
usage also covers the English semantic content of "fetus" and
"infant." Grammatically, *aulad* should pair with *bacche*, the plural
of *baccha*, but I heard the word *aulad* mostly used as a singular
noun. In my first standard reference for Hindi, I found the definition given above and did not think much of it. Later, though,
when I began sifting through my notes, interviews, and materials
gathered from popular literature and film, I realized that the term
appeared frequently, but not as I expected, and I decided that I
should look into the notion of *aulad* in more depth. In other dictionaries, I found more detailed definitions:

اولاد

aulad N.F. PL. children, descendants, offspring; progeny—*aulad-
e-inās* N.F. PL. daughters—*aulad-e-zūkoor* N.F. PL. sons—*halāl
ki aulad* N.F. PL. legitimate children well-behaved progeny—
nā<u>kh</u>a'laf aulad N.F. PL. unmannerly or good-for-nothing progeny [A.~ SING. valad]. (Qureshi and Haq 1999, 83)

اولاد

aulad, s.f. pl. (of *walad*), Children, descendants, offspring, issue,
progeny (usually constructed with a sing. verb): –*auladu'l-halāl*,
s.f. Legitimate children: –*aulad-e-anāsāl* or *inās*, s.f. Female
issue: –*aulad-e-zukūr*, Male issue: –*aulad-e-rishta-e-mustaqīma*,
s.f. Children in a direct line, lineal descendants: –*aulad-e-
sahīhu'n-nasab*, s.f. Legitimate children or issue (=*auladu'l-halāl*):
–*aulad-e-gair-sahīhu'n-nasab*, s.f. Illegitimate children or issue:
–*aulad-ki aulad*, s.f. Grandchildren: –*aulad-e-najību't-tarfain*,
s.f. Legitimate issue from both sides (paternal and maternal): –
aulad-e-nasabi, s.f. Legitimate issue (=*auladu'l-halāl*). (Platts 1977
[1884], 107)

The first definition comes from a contemporary Urdu-to-En-
glish dictionary published in Delhi. The second comes from *Platts'*
Dictionary of Urdu, Classical Hindi, and English, which was originally published in the nineteenth century but is still the standard

for quality and thoroughness as a reference work. According
to both definitions, *aulad* are not just children; they are specifically "progeny," a term that assumes biological paternity and
legal legitimacy. As these more detailed definitions point out,
aulad can be qualified (or marked) in a number of ways. Whether
these differences are evidence of historical change toward narrowing definitions of *aulad* or are indicative of the thoroughness
of the contemporary dictionary, or something else, remains an
unresolved historical matter. Narrowing of the acceptable categories since the 1800s would seem to follow a trend noted by
historians and anthropologists working on transformations of
marriage, kinship, and inheritance in different parts of India
(Bharadwaj 2016; Ramberg 2014; Sturman 2012; Sreenivas 2008).
Scholars have documented diverse, often hierarchically ranked
ways of accounting for partners and children, particularly sons,
in ancient Hindu texts and in local practice. A key example of
the creativity embodied in such texts and practices is the case
of *jogatis/devadasis* documented by Lucinda Ramberg in the
southern states of Karnataka and Maharashtra. Female-bodied
people identifying as women could structurally take on the responsibilities and privileges of sons in their natal households by
being dedicated/married to the goddess Yellamma as *jogatis/
devadasis*, instead of being married to a man (Ramberg 2014).
Many of these kinship categories and practices have been legally
limited or eliminated over time since the British colonial era,
including that of the *devadasi*. The marked categories of *aulad*
provided in dictionaries rarely appear in contemporary practice
in Uttar Pradesh, except in particular legal circumstances where
these details would be closely examined to determine the rights
of conflicting parties, such as in cases dealing with Islamic inheritance laws.

   In formal Urdu, the language of begetting defines a whole series of relationships. Begetting literally refers to "siring" a child
and focuses on the male contribution. The Arabic root comprised

of the letters v, l, and d, which Platts defines as "to beget" (Platts 1977 [1884], 1200), unites these concepts, linguistically speaking. From the v-l-d root come the words *wālid* (father); *wālida* (mother; feminine form of *wālid*); *wāliden* (parents); *walad* (son/offspring; singular, grammatically masculine); and *aulad* (plural, grammatically feminine). Apart from the term *aulad*, only Muslims in Lucknow generally use these "begetting" kinship terms, and their use may be contextual and stand alongside more intimate terms such as *ammi* (mummy) and *abba* (papa). Although defining these relationships is extremely relevant to legal matters such as inheritance, to be *aulad* is not simply to be an heir—a separate term, *wāris*, carries that meaning. The prefix *be-* in Urdu adds the meaning of "lack" or "without." To be *beaulad* (beaulād, adjective) is literally to be "without progeny" or childless; *beauladi* (noun) equates to the state or condition referred to somewhat awkwardly in scholarly literature in English as childlessness. A person who is *bewāris* (or *lawāris*, again, without-*wāris*) has no heir. All of these related terms that carry *aulad* are familiar and common to people living in Lucknow and are not only used by Muslims. In formal Hindi, the most common word for being childless is *santanhin* (santānhīn; progeny-without), a term that carries similar connotations of biological connection and breeding. Because the word *aulad* was used colloquially by people in Lucknow from different religious backgrounds, and occurred most frequently in speech, literature, and films, I focus on that term.

As I reflected on my fieldwork notes, I realized that mentions of *aulad* turned up often, but the varied meanings of *aulad* had to be unpacked in order to understand what was at stake for people suffering from infertility. For example, dictionary definitions gave only the slightest hint that *aulad* might refer to children of one sex or the other, but some women in Lucknow vehemently argued that only sons truly counted as *aulad*. Such variation in meanings led me to further questions: When was the existence of *aulad* ensured? Was the birth of a child, or of a son, on its own, sufficient for a married woman to avoid the suffering associated with being *beaulad*? Could women and their allies exercise their own agency and creativity to fulfill, approximate, or redefine these ideals about children to meet their own needs? And what obstacles might they face along the way?

CHILD DESIRE, THE VALUE OF CHILDREN, AND THE STAKES OF *AULAD*

For people who do not wish to create biological children, infertility can be a nonissue or even a desired condition. Indeed, it is a condition that many people in the contemporary world induce through the use of contraceptives, nonprocreative sex, and/ or abstinence at some point in their reproductive lives. Some fall into Arthur Greil and Julia McQuillan's (2010) category of people who might be classified as "infertile" but who instead see themselves as lacking in intent to produce a child. Others, as Kristin Wilson has argued, may see themselves as "not trying," or they might define their situations in other ways (2009, 2018). In other words, their inability to conceive or give birth to a child is not a matter of great anguish, pain, or suffering. Margarete Sandelowski has argued that infertility starts not with the inability to have a child but with the desire to have a child (Sandelowski 1993, 19, cited in Chase and Rogers 2001, 175). The element of desire for a child, with added cultural contours—such as a child produced through a particular method, with particular physical characteristics, gestated in a particular womb, and so on—presses people to seek out a child so long as that desire remains unfulfilled. After a long period of conflict over legitimate marriage, control of sexuality, and kinship in contemporary India, the "married body," as argued by Bharadwaj (2003, 1850) has largely been codified as the normative reproductive unit.[9] Biomedical ethical guidelines do not preclude others from using ARTs in attempts to procreate, but government regulations are moving toward restrictions on who may use these technologies in India. Adoption regulations are more stringent in terms of who may adopt children.

"Child desire," as a particular variety of yearning, is a phrase often found in works of demography and in studies about the "value of children." Many such surveys were conducted by population scientists around the world beginning in the 1970s and served as crucial tools of biopower (Foucault 1978). These surveys were often part of projects intended to understand cultural attitudes toward children with the objective of creating social change to reduce the number of births per woman, and to convince people in "developing" countries to embrace the small-family norm (no more than two or three children) (Arnold et al. 1975).[10] These studies often addressed such topics as how many children were wanted by a woman (or couple, or men and women separately) and what sex they were. In places like India, women reported having more children than they actually wanted, which supposedly indicated an unmet demand for contraceptive devices, and that they wanted more sons than daughters.

The "value of children," as reported from India, has been discussed in terms of "traditional" values such as continuing a family line (patrilineal, *vansh* or *khaandaan*), conducting funerary rituals and providing old-age support. The importance of children has also been assessed in terms of "emotional" values such as preventing loneliness or having someone to love and devote one's energies toward (Mishra et al. 2005; Sen and Drèze 1999, 172–75; Das Gupta 1995; Vlassoff 1990). The question of what value children might hold for people who did not have them but wanted to have them did not figure prominently in the rhetoric of the time. Malthusian fears about population growth, rather than relative levels of consumption of resources (Diamond 2008) or other ways of approaching the importance of the numerical size of human populations, figured prominently in studies of the time. These fears, which have not disappeared in subsequent decades, were reflected in popular books such as Paul Ehrlich's 1968 work *The Population Bomb*, which predicted massive human misery if births were not rapidly curbed.[11] In the 1960s, India's population numbered far less than the current (2019) estimate of 1.36 billion, second in the world only to China (World Bank 2019; Burke 2011).

In contemporary India, the contrasts of privilege and poverty are readily apparent in the day-to-day work of raising children. While some children study in elite English-language schools and are bathed and hand-fed by their mothers until they are eight or more, others wander the streets or work in fields ranging from dishwashing to embroidery. Privileged, wanted babies receive care in extreme measure, while unwanted babies—often female and/or presumed to have been born under scandalous conditions—are abandoned by the roadside or neglected to the point of death. Still others may be sold by their parents, or kidnapped and sold by others, for their potential as workers, including as sex workers (*In-Country* 2009; Ali and Thukral 2007; Pradhana 1997; Rozario 1988). That poor people do not love their children does not follow from these observations. For example, when asked by survey workers about the value of children, people in and around the city of Varanasi (in eastern Uttar Pradesh) placed a high value on children (Mishra et al. 2005, 165), even if the realities of everyday life made it difficult for people to actualize a level of care that would demonstrate to others that they valued their children. Still, surveys have often left out detailed considerations of the nuances of child desire: *Which* children are valued most and by whom? The question may seem a crass one, but it has great significance for a range of potential relatives evaluating their present conditions of life and the potential future lives they envision for themselves and their children.

The idea of child desire (*bacche ki chah*) has two main parts, the contours of which both bear consideration as being culturally particular ideas. The desire to have a child or children depends on specific understandings of the value of children, the characteristics of children, and the relationship between children and the families who raise them. In India, "desire" has often been constructed both as a force that keeps the world in motion and as a possible source of destruction. In North India, the idea of *nazar* or *kudrishti* (the gaze or evil eye) structures much talk about the dangerous nature of the desires harbored by people. Desire can "stick" to the person receiving the gaze, which can lead to illness or accidents and must be removed through ritual and/or guarded against by using talismans or other protective devices (Spiro 2005; Choudhry 1997; Nichter 1981; Maloney 1976).

When examining child desire as one part of reproductive desires in India, the question of agency also arises. Who desires a child? How do they communicate those desires? And whose desires take priority? From a cross-cultural perspective, possibilities include the state, ancestors, human bodies, people of all gender identities and sexual orientations, and people in various kin relationships to potential parents. Focusing on the desires of individuals, or of partners, is not sufficient to understand most lived experiences of reproduction in North India. To grasp the extent of women's autonomy (Bloom, Wypij, and Das Gupta 2001; Jejeebhoy and Sathar 2001; Das Gupta 1995) in reproduction, the roles played by the extended family, especially the mother-in-law, also need to be considered (Säävälä 1999; Jeffery and Jeffery 1996; Freed and Freed 1989). Put another way, whose desires matter and what does kinship do for people involved in reproduction? What sorts of culturally sanctioned practical kinship, workarounds, or *aankon ka parda* (strategically turning one's eyes away) might be used to approximate ideal reproduction? (Bourdieu 1990; Ramberg 2014).

In Uttar Pradesh, the desire for a child encompasses the desire to initiate a whole series of relationships, not only mother
and father but also maternal and paternal grandmother, maternal
and paternal grandfather, aunt (mother's sister, father's sister, father's brother's wife, mother's brother's wife), uncle (father's elder
brother, father's younger brother, mother's brother, father's sister's husband, mother's sister's husband), and other relationships
delineated by Hindi and Urdu. These specific relationships come
with intricate and specific expectations about obligations for residence, gift exchange, ritual roles, and affection. In North India,
the strongest distinctions between relations turn on whether they
are maternal or paternal relations and whether they are relatively
older or younger than one's parents or parents-in-law (for example, see Vatuk 1982 and Turner 1975). New relationships initi-
ated through the addition of a new child often include redefining
friends, neighbors, and relatives as aunts, uncles, brothers, sisters,
grandparents, and so forth. Now out of fashion in some circles,
there are long-held traditions in North India of calling women by
different names depending on their stage of life, such that they
may be known by their given names for a short period before
marriage. After marriage, given names would yield to "wife of so-
and-so," then "mother of so-and-so." Even when such conventions
fall out of use, they may be invoked in a joking way as a reminder
of village practices or used in particular ritual contexts.

The meanings of a child go beyond what a child means for
the father and mother, and beyond the dictates of specific ritual
events, such as the need for a son to perform funerary rituals.
Children are defined differently depending on their particular
relationship with the household. The children of daughters and
the children of sons belong to different households, since the
primary "home" of a married daughter is ideally with her in-
laws, and her children are supposed to belong there, while the
children of sons remain part of their fathers' households. This

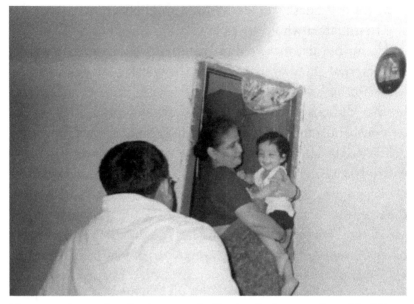

Figure 1.3. A grandmother's care and affection for her grandson. *Nani ji* and *nati* (maternal grandmother and grandson). (Photo by author.)

sense of affiliation pertains not only to children's membership in a lineage but also to the attribution of responsibility for the care and expense associated with their upbringing. The differences between grandchildren are reflected in Hindi/Urdu, with the terms *nati* (nātī) and *natin* (nātin) referring to the son and daughter of one's daughter, and the terms *pota* (pōtā) and *poti* (pōtī) referring to the son and daughter of one's son. A similar system applies for referring to the relationships denoted by the English terms "niece" and "nephew," with the terms *bhanja* (bhānja) and *bhanji* (bhānji) identifying the son and daughter of one's sister, and *bhatija* (bhatījā) and *bhatiji* (bhatījī) identifying the son and daughter of one's brother.[12]

I do not say that Hindi/Urdu speakers parcel out or measure their affection toward particular children based on their relationship category but rather that the emotional baggage and structural expectations attached to particular relationships mean that, for example, grandparents with several *natis* may still yearn for a *pota*, or that those with a *pota* may still feel the lack of a *poti*. Those who expect that their sons might continue to live with them after marriage might also expect to care for, and to be cared for by, their sons' children more intensely than by their daughters' children. Cultural preferences for sons may well influence these feelings and the ways the older generation attempts to influence the reproductive lives of the younger generation, whether or not they actually reside together. In small families, which have become much more prevalent in the last half century—as the average number of births per woman has been more than halved across India—the stakes of each child's fertility are much higher, if family members understand that the continuity of the family can be ensured only through the birth of children who can be classified as *aulad*, and direct their desires toward attaining that ideal. Exactly which children can fit into this category depends on context, with some informants arguing that any child brought into a family through the normal course of marriage and pregnancy could count, while others contended that only male children can count as *aulad*. In the case of male children, they are then all *aulad* for their parents, but from the grandparents' perspective, only the sons of sons fall into that category. Other culturally sanctioned ways of fulfilling these ideals in North India, particularly among households without sons, include recruiting a *ghar jamai* (ghar jamaī), a daughter's husband who shifts alliance toward her natal family. This practice has low cultural value but is a possibility and will be addressed in more detail in chapter 4. Other intriguing models exist on the margins of South Asian practice, such as the transformation of *jogatis*, women dedicated to the goddess in South India (described by Ramberg 2014) into structural sons, making their children into kin that might fit the model of *aulad* or *pota* (as the children of a son), but Ramberg argues that this practice is becoming uncommon and may disappear.

Much scholarly work and government policy in India has studied and attempted to intervene in the phenomenon of son preference. Research documents son preference as one reason why families might continue to have children beyond their desired family size. Such studies have attempted to explain the neglect, abandonment, and killing of female children and the selective abortion of female fetuses as being rooted in a preference for sons, a preference that varies in intensity to some extent by religious background and dowry practices of particular caste and religious groups (Patel 2007a provides a good introduction and specific case studies). Apart from biological relation—which most people take as a given unless difficulties arise—the sex of the child is the most frequently mentioned object of desire, with most people wishing for at least one son and then, perhaps, a daughter. Other desired traits in children may be skin color, weight, health status, or quantity of hair. Here and there, in conversations and in public discourse, hints about the stakes of child desire and its fulfillment emerge.

For married couples, infertility presents a crisis in their understanding of the normal course of a marriage and a unique chance to consider the potential composition of their families. The harassment of childless women by their in-laws and neighbors is a common theme in fertility studies. In my study, women with and without children discussed this theme in conversations about infertility and the options available to deal with it. However, in interviews I conducted during fieldwork with women who were currently undergoing treatment for infertility in public hospitals in Lucknow, which I examine in greater depth in the next two chapters, a more complex picture of familial relations in infertility came into focus. So did a variety of perspectives on the value of children, the le-

gitimacy of relationships between parents and children, and
the possibilities of creating novel family ties under the veil
of secrecy, rather than openly challenging societal norms
about appropriate reproduction. Through their negotiations,
actions, and choices as they navigated infertility treatment,
women undergoing biomedical infertility treatment were attempting to quietly revolutionize the distribution of power,
intimacies, and resources within their households. Yet, they
strove to maintain the appearance of conforming to conventional reproductive ideals. The goal of maintaining secrecy
about some aspects of infertility treatment, while disclosing
details necessary to recruiting help with the logistics of treatment, was, for many women, key to pursuing children through
biomedical treatment.

CLINICAL MANAGEMENT OF THE DESIRES
OF FAMILY AND "SOCIETY"

Women I interviewed in infertility clinics in Lucknow often
pointed to prejudices against married, childless women that de-
monize them as grasping victims of desire who may—intention-
ally or otherwise—bring harm to others. Some women expressed
the specific desire to have a son, while others argued that for
people "in this condition" any child, male or female, would suf-
fice. Some of them were receiving intrauterine insemination with
donor sperm, which they saw as a less legitimate way of conceiving, but they preferred it to adoption. Most saw adoption as a
last resort, clearly inferior to producing a child with some sort
of biological tie, whether imagined through genes, "blood," or
pregnancy.

"Samaj men rahna hai to samaj ke hisaab se rahna paṛta hai."
"If one has to live in society, then one has to live according to
society's ways."[13]

Seema

A Hindu woman, Seema, from a small city about eighty kilometers from Lucknow reported that her husband of nine years usually accompanied her to the infertility clinic where she had been undergoing treatment for a year, even though she was having treatment with donor sperm because testing had revealed a male-factor infertility problem. She said, "It was a deficiency in my husband. His semen (water/*paani*) was useless. At home no one else knows that they use another's [another man's semen]. My in-laws say to go and try [literally "show"] somewhere else." Her narration of the family history, in which both of her husband's elder brothers had children only after six to eight years of marriage, suggests a family history of male-factor infertility problems. This couple had also considered adoption, but only if the treatment was unsuccessful, and only if everyone at home agreed. According to Seema, "We thought it's possible this year we'll get some benefit, and we may not be forced to take someone else's [child] [note the use of subjunctive/conditional verb in both clauses]." The hospital had required both partners to sign their consent (*ki hum sehmat hain,* that we agree) for the use of donor sperm in their treatment. Seema said that her husband "had to think about it," but in the end, he accepted this course of treatment.

According to the head nurse in a large government infertility unit, with whom I chatted frequently before the day's round of treatment began or at the end of her shift, consent from both partners was absolutely required before donor sperm could be used in infertility treatment. She did not know for sure, however, where the donor sperm came from, other than from the laboratory. She suggested that samples given by other men for diagnostic testing may be used for donor insemination, but no one had ever asked about the origin of the donor sperm. Most of the time, patients agreed to use donor sperm, but both husbands and wives could and did refuse this treatment—it is not the case that only husbands rejected treatment with donor sperm. She also argued that, among the patients, religion was never a stated reason for rejecting a particular treatment. The prospect of demonstrating to people in the surrounding society (*samaj men dikhana*) that a birth had taken place in their household and presenting the child as their own—which the nurse seemed to see as a deceptive act—would motivate some patients to accept donor sperm. The use of donor sperm could easily be concealed from other family members and from neighbors and "society" in general, and therefore presented a pragmatic approach to solving infertility that many, though not all, couples could accept. In cases where couples accepted donor sperm, living according to the ways of family and "society" may not have been as crucial as *appearing* to do so.

Women's expressions of child desire in clinics varied. Some women, although they were clearly investing significant amounts of their time and financial resources in treatment, questioned the need for children in general and the necessity of raising children conceived and born within the conventional configuration of gametes and wombs, albeit with the help of the technological assistance provided by the clinic. "Society" (*samaj*) in a general sense appeared in women's narratives frequently as the enforcer of pronatalism, the promoter of motherhood, and one of the major reasons why childless married women suffered. One Hindu woman, who had been married for ten years without a child, explained that "they don't say it to your face, but they say it behind your back. . . . One has to do it [have a child] for society. These days, children don't even do anything special for their parents. Children create difficulties, too." Several other Hindu women added that mothers-in-law have the right to, and do, comment on the fertility status of their daughters-in-law.

While some women focused intense attention on the views of outsiders, others were especially keen to discuss relationships within their families. According to these women, fertility status has a significant impact on relationships within the household and clarifies that the desire for children is not limited only to couples of childbearing age but that extended families and even other children in the family may also express these wishes and put pressure on women of childbearing age, and perhaps on their husbands, as well. Infertility, as demonstrated in women's narratives, can disrupt established paths for daughters-in-law to increase their status in their marital households. It may also promote husband-wife solidarity against other household members, which wives might see as a good thing, to the chagrin of other family members. Two figures appeared most frequently in women's narratives about dealing with infertility: mothers-in-law and husbands. Some women experienced tension in their home relations because of their childlessness, while others were able to successfully make use of their relationships in order to facilitate their treatment.

Several themes recurred in our discussions, including the conflicting role of mothers-in-law and the support offered by husbands. Despite differences in marriage practices among Hindus and Muslims, I found that women expressed common themes about household dynamics that did not map neatly onto religious division. Some women experienced tension in their relationships with members of their marital household that contributed to their seeking infertility treatment. These women commonly reported that their mothers-in-law (*saas* or *saasu ma*) wanted to find another wife for their sons, one who would be able to produce children. However, in nearly as many cases as women criticized their mothers-in-law for trying to persuade their sons to remarry, they—often in the same breath—praised their husbands for refusing to listen to their mothers. Husbands,

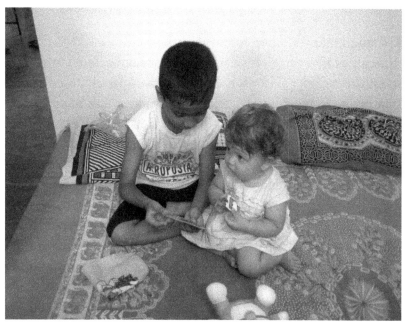

Figure 1.4. Siblings, cousins, and close friends celebrate the bonds of protection and affection between brothers and sisters on holidays such as Raksha Bandhan with gifts, sweets, and *rakhi*s that sisters commonly tie on their brothers' wrists. (Photo by author.)

in their wives' words, supported their wives and accompanied them on trips to clinics and hospitals for treatment. Some husbands tried to persuade their wives to give up treatment and be happy as they were, without children, or to consider adopting a child. In these conversations about relationships with supportive husbands, the gendered dynamics for women in dealing with infertility in the North Indian context began to become clear. Yet they were not as I had expected. Women were highly likely to defend their husbands and to emphasize their own desire for children, their "own" children, over the wishes of their husbands.

Manju and Shaheen

Although many women found that their childless state created difficulties in managing relationships at home, some were able to enlist the help of household members to facilitate infertility treatment. They would disclose some information to particular members but keep certain details of the treatment secret. By strategically sharing some information about their treatment, they were able to recruit other women in the household to help with chores while they traveled to the clinic, to secure money for treatment costs or company for the journey, or to fend off comments from neighbors about their frequent trips away from home. Those who came to the clinic from outside of Lucknow often recruited other women in the household to care for other children they might have while they stayed in Lucknow for up to ten days of treatment.

A Hindu woman named Manju, originally from Kanpur, said that her mother-in-law was very good, and would send her for treatment even when she didn't feel like going to the clinic, while her father-in-law bore the cost of treatment without complaint. Despite the strong role her in-laws played in her treatment, Manju focused on her eight-year-old daughter as the main force behind her treatment, saying that she would like to have a brother for her daughter, so that she would be able to tie a *rakhi* (an ornamented string bracelet) on someone on holidays like Raksha Bandhan, which celebrates the special relationship between brothers and sisters. Manju's focus was not simply on having a son but on creating the special relationship between siblings that she wanted to provide to her daughter. A Muslim woman, Shaheen, from Lucknow, told me about her wish to have a *joRa* (pair) of children. She had an eight-year-old son, but no other children, and she cited her son's desire to have a brother or sister—saying that he cried whenever anyone mentioned a brother or sister to him—as a major reason for her to undergo infertility treatment.

WHY PETS ARE NOT AN OPTION

Many of my early conversations about my research project with South Asian people, inside and beyond infertility clinics, and with South Asians in the United States, have touched on the topic of pets as a substitute for children. South Asians I have known in the United States have found it laughable that the question "How many children do you have?" should be answered with "We have two dogs."[14] Theories of child desire that have to do with structural considerations in joint families demonstrate expectations that daughters-in-law benefit from the birth of children, especially sons, and that children enliven multigenerational households, whether they reside together or not.

Rama, Razia, and Gunja

For women in infertility clinics in Lucknow, family dynamics were certainly a crucial consideration in their quests for children, and they pertained not only to husbands and wives but to relationships of brothers, sisters, parents, and in-laws as well. Women linked family discord to the absence of children, and hoped that by successfully obtaining children, they could bring harmony to the household. Rama argued that a lack of children in the household caused fighting among its members. Razia from Faizabad said that whenever arguments broke out in her household, her father-in-law would point out the absence of children and the threat to the continuance of the family lineage. No one suggested that the presence of a loving animal could fill the void felt among household members. In any case, the dog is used as a favorite term of abuse much more frequently than it is embraced as a family member in South Asia. Not just any child qualifies culturally to fill this void, either. Ideas about blood and belonging come into play, and the sex and physical capacity of a child are also relevant considerations. Women undergoing infertility treatments generally expressed some flexibility about making families. Still, they varied in their willingness to consider adopting strategies for obtaining children that carried the risk of stigma or rejection from other family members or "society."

Emotional arguments about the affective relationships between people and the necessity of children went beyond personal desires to experience pregnancy or motherhood, and beyond childbearing as a means of creating or salvaging a husband-wife bond. Gunja, whose husband worked in the Persian Gulf and only came home to India periodically, felt that she had learned much about the value of children from her own experiences. She had been married while she was still completing her bachelor's degree, and she and her husband had used birth control during the first three years of their marriage. She contrasted that time, when they were always anxious that her period not be delayed, with the present, when they wished it would not arrive. She said that her mother had passed away after her marriage, waiting to become a grandmother (*nani*, nānī), and so had her father-in-law (*sasur*). She argued that her child would be a king (*raja*, implies "son") both in her natal home (*maike*) and her in-laws' home (*sasural*). "The child is not for my happiness (*khushi*), it's for the happiness of others. It will certainly bring a smile to my face, but it will also bring a smile to everyone else's face as well."

In the familial politics of fertility, which can be extended to include the specter of neighborhood gossip, another aspect of the fertility-infertility dialectic described by Inhorn (1994) emerges, in that many places where high rates of fertility prevail, high rates of infertility, as well as high infant and child mortality, can also be found. The contrast between expectations and stereotypes of families with many children and the reality of infertility, whether primary or secondary, can heighten the distress felt by people seeking solutions to their infertility. In families and locales with an abundance of children, particularly many children who are ill-treated or disregarded by their parents, the sting of a lack of children felt by people unable to fulfill their desires for them can increase, especially for women who rarely move beyond the confines of their own home or neighborhood. The abundance of children has the potential to either alleviate the pain associated with childlessness or otherwise unfulfilled reproductive aspiration— "there are other children around, so what does it matter?"—or to exacerbate the pain associated with their child desire—"there are other children around, why not mine?"

Beyond the larger picture of inheritance and power, the small daily ways that extended families deal with distributing the care of children, of affection, and of rights within the household can significantly influence infertility experiences, as demonstrated by Qudsia baji's narration of her experiences of coexisting with her in-laws while waiting for *aulad*. Whether the waiting is due to infertility problems or not, the emotional effects of family members' comments about women's fertility status can significantly impact their self-image and perception of their value in the household. The importance of and meanings of children extend beyond the psychological implications of in/fertility for individual women or married partners. Reproductive politics take on particular significance in the context of extended patriarchal families and have strong potential implications for the division of power, resources, and affection within those families. The desire to produce particular sorts of children within the context of a joint marital home can lead to competition or cooperation, depending on the relationships within the family, and depending on the success of particular members in fulfilling their reproductive desires.

NOTES

1. All personal names are given as pseudonyms. *Baji* is a general term in Urdu that means "sister" or "elder sister" and is often used as a term of respect. The Urdu word *Aapa* also means "elder sister" and is used in simi-

lar ways to *baji*. See also Singh 2017. Quotations in this chapter come from
interviews I conducted in Lucknow in infertility clinics and meetings in
various spaces from 2005 to 2007. This chapter also includes excerpts from
and references to my fieldnotes composed during the same time.

2. Lyrics, translation, and link to recording: See the entry at Filmy
Quotes, Baabul Ki Duayein Leti Ja https://www.filmyquotes.com
/songs/3611, accessed April 10, 2022. Scenes from film *Neel Kamal*
performed by Mohammed Rafi: https://www.youtube.com/watch
?v=K8YBicA7HWE and https://www.youtube.com/watch?v=-8Ke
BXm6gYU. Recent remake by Sonu Nigam at https://www.youtube.com
/watch?v=o3jFsxJSJ9s accessed June 15, 2021.

3. Lyrics, translation, and link to recording: See the entry at Filmy
Quotes, Baabul Ki Duayein Leti Ja https://www.filmyquotes.com
/songs/3611, accessed April 10, 2022. Scenes from film *Neel Kamal*
performed by Mohammed Rafi: https://www.youtube.com/watch?v
=K8YBicA7HWE and https://www.youtube.com/watch?v=-8KeB
Xm6gYU. Recent remake by Sonu Nigam at https://www.youtube.com
/watch?v=o3jFsxJSJ9s accessed 15 June 2021.

4. For a detailed examination of the issues involved in gift exchange,
marriage, and hierarchy in India, see, for example, work by Louis Dumont
(Dumont [1967] 1980), responses to Dumont (Khare 2006), and ethnographies of exchange in India (Gregory 1997; Parry 1994; Raheja 1988).

5. Full song: https://www.youtube.com/watch?v=nqydfARGDh4.
Lyrics and English translation: https://www.filmyquotes.com/songs/975,
accessed June 17, 2021.

6. http://www.youtube.com/watch?v=AgiMhAH2jj8&feature=
related, accessed November 10, 2010.

7. http://www.youtube.com/watch?v=AgiMhAH2jj8&feature=
related, accessed November 10, 2010.

8. https://www.hotstar.com/in/tv/sasural-genda-phool/467, accessed
June 13, 2022.

9. See Ramberg (2014), Sreenivas (2008), and Sturman (2012) for more
on legal reforms in relation to historical transformations of women's status
through marriage, landholding, and so on.

10. Information on some of the organizations involved in the production and funding of studies of this sort can be found at the Population
Council, http://www.popcouncil.org; Demographic and Health Surveys,
http://www.measuredhs.com; and Population Reference Bureau, http://
www.prb.org.

11. A full discussion of the critique of that book and the massive expenditure on programs created in that era to control population is beyond the scope of this book. For more information, see Diamond (2008), Hartmann (1987), and the Population and Development Program records archived at the Sophia Smith Collection of Women's History at Smith College.

12. For further analysis of Hindi/Urdu kinship terminology, see James Turner (1975) and Sylvia Vatuk (1982).

13. Fieldnotes November 5, 2007.

14. I especially thank Anand Dwivedi for his insights on this issue in extended conversations.

TWO

PRELUDES TO *AULAD*

Making Mothers

Whatever happens, the one who has nobody . . . To become
a mother is the most important job. Outsiders say, "that poor
lady." The one who doesn't have any children learns what their
importance is.

> —Sikh woman undergoing infertility treatment, group
> conversation, Lucknow infertility clinic, 2007

PRESCRIBING MOTHERHOOD

Dr. Kapoor

On July 4, 2005, I sat in the room designated for patient education sessions at a private infertility clinic in Lucknow, awaiting
the arrival of the head physician and public face of the clinic, Dr.
Kapoor.[1] The room had clean, sterile-looking white walls and
chairs arranged as if in preparation for a public lecture. A table
and a whiteboard were covered with acronyms of procedures
and figures—from just over ten dollars to more than two hundred dollars—that appeared to be the cost of each procedure. A
diagram titled "The Triangle of Infertility: S/O/UT," a formula
for explaining how the sperm, ovum, and uterus meet to create
the fetus pictured in the center of the triangle, completed the

academic atmosphere of the space. Posters with English titles such as "The Journey of Human Life," and a few with Hindi text, "IVF kya hai?, ICSI kya hai?" ("What is IVF? What is ICSI?" [*in vitro fertilization* and *intracytoplasmic sperm injection*]) dotted the walls. The television at the front of the room played a video that described procedures used in biomedical infertility treatment. Several couples, and a few groups including an older woman, were also waiting for the physician's arrival. These groups waited, files in hand, to be called for consultation with the clinic's staff. In this elaborate prelude to the head physician's arrival, we were all treated to cold drinks and snacks.

Finally, the physician swept into the room, her considerable presence enhanced by her height, solid build, and the deference she received from those in attendance and from her staff. She promptly launched forth into explanations about her clinic, the procedures offered, and the length of time involved. Frank in her discussion, which she termed, "face to face, bilateral talks,"[2] she seemed focused on dispelling rumors and not fostering delusions about infertility treatments and the prospects that these treatments would lead to the birth of a child. Even in the best international clinics, she emphasized, the success rate does not exceed 40 percent. In infertility in India, she said, effects of tuberculosis on the reproductive system and the absence of sperm (azoospermia) are quite common, in contrast with many other countries where assisted reproductive technologies such as in vitro fertilization are readily available. To undergo treatment, some people would need to commit to significant changes in their lifestyle, including losing weight, stopping smoking, and cutting back on other common hazards that could affect their fertility. A lack of commitment would signal the absence of desire for a child. Still, hidden factors (*chupi hui chizen*) could interfere in the scientific procedures—treatment would not include magic (*jadu*, jādū).

While explaining the scientific procedures and the economic investment required for treatment in her facility, Dr. Kapoor ruminated on the phenomenon of infertility. In her view, infertility is not a disease (*rog*) but a "natural handicap"; that is, infertility in and of itself does not threaten the physical life of a human being. However, societal and familial factors intersect to influence lived experiences of infertility, which can be quite difficult for the people involved. In this initial group session, she also offered specific advice about how to negotiate family dynamics during infertility treatment. Her recommendations included carefully considering the benefits and harms (*fayda/nuksan*) of involving family members in treatment, including as potential gamete donors, before taking any such step. She accepted the idea that partners might hide aspects of their treatment from their families but rejected the notion that the spouses might conceal anything from each other in infertility treatment.

Dr. Kapoor's social analysis was keen and echoes theoretical contributions by social scientists on the nature of infertility (Sandelowski and de Lacey 2002; Sandelowski 1993; Greil 1991). Infertility may never be discovered, nor experienced as a problem, by people whose life course does not include attempts to conceive and bear children, and it may cause no pain in and of itself. Still, the status of infertility as an affliction may range through many different experiences of pain, loss, anger, and possible bodily harm, depending on the social and cultural context in which people attempt to cope with infertility (van Balen and Inhorn 2002, 5–7). While Dr. Kapoor advocated for couples' quests for children, she also encouraged them to consider alternatives to obtaining a genetically related child through the use of assisted reproductive technologies available at her clinic.

Dr. Kapoor argued that not having a child would turn couples into *sadhus* (religious figures, renouncers of worldly attachments) and—as she put it—finish off their motivation, their family's progression, and society's progression. Even though, in her opinion, many members of their extended family would secretly wish them to remain childless because of matters of inheritance, and even though the government would not reimburse them for infertility treatment, she encouraged them to continue on some path toward obtaining a child, to fulfill the dictum of another of the posters on the classroom wall, which read, "Motherhood: The Right of Every Woman." Dr. Kapoor made clear that her clinic also provided counseling and advice for couples about how to proceed with child adoption at that time or at any time during their treatment. She also advised couples to consider treatment costs and not to sacrifice their ability to raise a future child through the pursuit of its birth. In short, she encouraged couples to pursue a life that included children, and although her business as an infertility specialist included the provision of many types of treatment that promised to fulfill (or to give the appearance of fulfilling) cultural ideals about procreation, she asked couples to think carefully about the long-term implications of this investment, given the likelihood of success and the long-term financial commitment involved in raising a child.

I know of no place in the world that lacks cultural ideals about parenting. North India certainly has an abundance of ideologies about parenthood and, in particular, about the importance of becoming a mother. In this chapter, I examine these ideals and their implications for fertility and infertility experiences by focusing on representations of mothers, motherhood, and mothering in popular media, by medical professionals, and by my interlocutors in Lucknow. These perspectives are critical to understanding the dilemmas faced by women suffering from infertility and reproductive loss when they consider the perspectives of "society" (samaj), which they often cited as a significant source of pressure and discontent about their unfulfilled reproductive aspirations. The definitions of and respect accorded to mothers, specifically in the North Indian context, shape the aspirations of women to become mothers by particular methods, and preferably not by others. Tulsi Patel has argued that fertility and motherhood are critical to women's survival in India (2007b, 37–38), which others have supported by referring to old-age security and emotional contentment while emphasizing the cultural importance of producing sons, which eventually leads to attaining relative security as a mother-in-law with sons' wives to care for them (Vlassoff 1990; Bumiller 1990; Das Gupta 1995; Dyson and Moore 1983). This emphasis on motherhood can be seen as another way of representing child desire and as part of the overarching frame of reproductive desires through the idiom of the particular mother-child relationship and with special reference to the women who mother, rather than the children they nurture.

Popular representations of motherhood and historical examples demonstrate some expansiveness in understandings of mothers, motherhood, and appropriate pairings of mothers and children. Yet, rankings of the value of particular types of mothering do emerge and influence women's perceptions of the best ways to become mothers. The increasing availability of assisted reproductive technologies helps to reinforce such hierarchies and encourages women to put off decisions either to pursue motherhood through ways other than giving birth or to accept a life without children of one's own. In these representations, unfulfilled reproductive desire emerges as a significant threat to women's well-being and to the smooth conduct of relationships in society.

IDENTIFYING AND EVALUATING MOTHERS
AND "MOTHERLY AFFECTION"

If you need to find out the value of a mother, find out from an orphan.
Ma ki qadar o qimat malum karni ho to kisi yateem se malum karo.[3]

—Farha Yasmeen, student at Karamat Hussain
Muslim Girls' Post-Graduate College,
Lucknow (2004–05), in the school magazine

In the previous chapter, I stressed the centrality of *aulad* as a culturally specific idea of progeny to women's attainment of

status within their marital homes. Many of my informants argued that not just any child would fulfill the criteria of *aulad*,
thereby creating parents' legitimate status as full adults and
"real" relatives to the child. Here, I examine this theme from a
different perspective by focusing on the messages women seeking to become mothers get about the appropriate ways to pursue
that goal. Dr. Kapoor's story from her patient education class
explores the possibility that women can achieve the status of
mother without giving birth themselves and without reproducing the culturally expected model of husband and wife physically
bound together in the form of a child created through the union
of their gametes. At the same time that Dr. Kapoor facilitated
the appearance of conventional childbirth using assisted reproductive technologies, she also pressed for the value of the act of
mothering, regardless of biological connection. In her presentation, this suggestion came across as transgressive of societal
norms, a transgression provoked by childlessness and induced by
infertility.

Ideologies of motherhood appear throughout many North Indian popular culture sources, from specialists like Dr. Kapoor
to media such as magazines, news, television, movies, and more.
These sources raise and address a variety of questions, such as
whether a mother who gives birth has greater worth and more
rights regarding a child than a woman who raises a child she did
not give birth to—and the consequences of separating a woman
who has given birth from her child. In each consideration of
mothers, the concept of *ma ki mamta* (mā kī mamtā, motherly
affection), plays a crucial role in understanding the stakes of becoming a mother. "*Mata* is usually a potential or actual mother.
Mother, motherlike (*mattravata*) and motherliness (*mattratva*)
are general categories of reference and description that are included in this social usage of the term. Thus, married but childless women and old unmarried women may be either addressed
or referred to as *mata-ji*. The usage is justified by seeing these
women as potential or metaphorical mothers; they may be seen

as a mother or motherlike, and in turn these women may also be motherly without actually being mothers" (Khare 1982, 156–60).

Social pressure to become a mother in the highest-prestige fashion, by giving birth to a child (preferably a son), is significant, and the potential results of not attaining this status can be dangerous both for a woman and those around her. Nonbirthing mothers are represented in popular culture, but most of my informants were skeptical of their acceptance and prestige. The level of acceptance may change in the context of expanded options for infertility treatment in contemporary India, including assisted reproductive technologies, and of popular attitudes toward child adoption. Women who marry men with children from a previous marriage and care for their husband's children, known as *sauteli* mothers (sautelī mā), get roundly abused in popular culture, much like the evil stepmother in the Cinderella story.

Other types of mothering relationships may be more or less readily accepted, although metaphorical attributions of motherliness are more likely to be considered acceptable than adoptive or foster relationships, based on the secrecy that generally surrounds the formation of such bonds. Indian media outlets give extensive news coverage to famous adoptive parents. For example, in 2006 and 2007, celebrities who had adopted children, such as Brad Pitt and Angelina Jolie, Madonna, and actress and former Miss Universe Sushmita Sen, figured prominently in entertainment and lifestyle sections of English and vernacular newspapers. In conversations during fieldwork, women, infertile or not, repeatedly emphasized adoption as a last resort when all other methods for obtaining a child had failed.

"WHAT ABOUT US?": INFERTILITY AND THE FUTURE

A small pamphlet published by the Population Council (Population Council 2002) reminds me of the politics of seeing, or otherwise sensing, reproductive disruption. In small text at the top of the cover is the question "What about Us?" This short but powerful question is followed by the subtitle "Bringing Infertility into Reproductive Health Care." The rest of the cover shows a sepia-toned photograph of an obviously pregnant Indian woman. She is wearing a printed sari made of synthetic material, not silk or cotton, and a sari blouse with puffed sleeves reminiscent of early-1990s fashion. Her jewelry is simple: glass bangles rather than gold; modest "small tops" earrings; a short black-and-gold beaded necklace and pendant called a *mangalsutra* that indicates her status as a married woman. A plain largish round bindi placed on her forehead, between her eyes where her "third eye" would be (according to Hindu mythology), suggests that she is Hindu. She does not face the camera but smiles just a little as she rests one hand above and one below her generous belly. The cast of sunlight on her face and clothing suggests that she is gazing out a window as she anticipates the arrival of her baby. She is the sole focus of the photograph; anyone else with a stake in the pregnancy remains outside the camera's view.

The publication describes efforts by the Population Council and other nongovernmental organizations to expand family-planning programs around the world. Notably, the stated aim of the expansion, a new venture, is to include people suffering from infertility. Historically, for countries accused of overpopulation like India, "family planning" meant reducing the number of births and increasing the time between births, rather than increasing fertility. The woman in the photo is not mentioned in the text that follows, so readers are left to wonder about her story. Does she represent an ideal of contentment in pregnancy? Or is she the picture of anticipated motherhood that women suffering their inability to birth children dream of? Does she represent the success of expanded "family planning" services in India? Readers are left to ponder the particulars of her story, the other people who might be anticipating the birth of her child, and the outcome of that pregnancy.

While studying the politics of reproduction in families and the nation-state in India, I found a vast literature on fertility and long histories of "family-planning" projects directed toward reducing the number of births. I became curious about the experiences of people for whom achieving conception and birth was either impossible or very difficult. Initially, I found only anecdotal evidence about the meanings of infertility in studies about high fertility and relatively few perspectives on cultural understandings of infertility or appropriate ways of resolving it. In the field, however, I found that understandings of the nature of children and the appropriate ways of creating relationships among children, parents, and members of the extended family are major factors that shape popular conceptions about infertility and suitable ways of overcoming a perceived lack of children.

Studies of various aspects of fertility in India have mentioned in passing the plight of infertile women, the degree to which they are ridiculed, seen as unfortunate creatures who at best inspire sadness, and at worst may use magic to steal away the children of others in order to get their own. In her study of fertility behavior in a village in Rajasthan, Western India, Tulsi Patel reported that barrenness was seen as a curse and a disgrace, but that it was highly gendered, with childless women suffering much more social stigma and psychological disturbance than childless men (1994, 78–79, 220–23). Sarah Pinto also described the danger to others posed by women whose reproductive lives had gone awry, especially to women and children:

> The overwhelming power of longing for a child characterizes figures imagined as most threatening: infertile women, witches, the *churel*. . . . Consumed by desire, they are pushed to consume the placenta, itself a place of leftover longing, receptacle of desire fulfilled, by eating or bewitching it, to "grab" the child, sap its life force. Briggs noted that in Awadh magical use of the placenta/cord taps the reproductive potential of the *mother*, her "gift of fertility" (1920, 60), having effect on the child: "If a woman eat

[a piece of the cord], the child will die, but she will obtain children." (Pinto 2008, 93–94)

Fantastic stories attributing misfortunes of infertility and child
death to ghosts and other supernatural forces certainly circulate in
many parts of India, but the effects of infertility on women are often much more concretely rooted in the conduct of their everyday
lives. Infertile women may be excluded from auspicious religious
and/or ritual occasions, or they may exclude themselves because of
their own perception of social stigma or of their own inauspicious-
ness. Pinto's work highlights the issue of desire and the danger that
women's desire for children can pose to others in the community
when left unfulfilled. Child desire, and especially the desire for
sons, is a force feared by those who have successfully achieved their
reproductive goals. Parents often attempt to shield their children
from such dangers by applying black marks of *kajal* (kohl), using
protective amulets called *taaviz*, or carrying out other ritual actions to avert or remove the evil eye (*buri nazar* or *kudrishti*).

In India, culturally speaking, infertility is a disaster. Infertility
threatens family continuity and tenuous attempts to influence the
future. For many people, not having children means not achieving peace. People suffering from infertility search for alternative
ways of obtaining children that can meet the culturally accepted
notions of being one's "own" (*apna*, apna), exemplified in Hindi/
Urdu by the term *aulad*. The acceptance of alternative strategies
for family formation fundamentally depends on cultural norms
for establishing legitimate kinship ties and, thereby, the ability
of people suffering from infertility to claim a child or children
as their "own." Across India, involuntary childlessness threatens
couples' potential to attain full personhood as adult members
of society and as full members of their kin networks. Infertility is not a life-threatening disorder when defined as a medical
condition rooted in the individual biological body. However,
childlessness brought on by infertility threatens social relations,

social status, and family honor. For young brides in the patrilocal and patrilineal kinship systems found throughout most of North India, this threat is particularly acute. Women who do not fulfill fertility expectations face social difficulties, potentially including divorce or dowry threats directed toward the wife's parents and siblings in her natal household (Unisa 1999; Patel 1994; Mandelbaum 1974). Without strong retirement or elder-care programs in place, childlessness can also pose a threat to health and safety in old age. The question "What about us?" encapsulates the desires, hopes, and fears contained within visions of the future people suffering from infertility might create.

One morning amid my fieldwork, I picked up the local edition of the *Times of India* to find a short news item about a young woman named Rasoolan, who had been hospitalized with burns all over her body after an incident at her in-laws' place. The case pertains to a Muslim family in the area of Kanpur, about fifty miles away from Lucknow. Rasoolan's uncle Mustaqeem accused Rasoolan's in-laws of trying to kill Rasoolan because she had not conceived a child during four years of marriage to a professional driver. Rasoolan's experiences can only be reconstructed from past conversations and reflections by her relatives, as she had been effectively silenced by the alleged crime. Reports of young women being burnt in their marital homes are far from uncommon in North India, but they are usually labeled as "dowry deaths," crimes in which in-laws' demands for dowry in the form of cash or other items eventually leads to a breakdown in intimate relationships and an "accident" at the kitchen stove. The storyline is familiar, but the cited reason is less so. Although nothing is proven in the article, the failure to conceive as a motive for attempting to dispose of a daughter-in-law fits into commonly held perceptions about the importance of children and the potential dangers of not producing children in North India. There is no question about the reasons why Rasoolan had not conceived a child. Regardless of any diagnosis a fertility specialist—medical, spiritual, or other—might give about the etiology of the problem, Rasoolan bore the consequences of infertility (*Times of India*, 2007, 6; Grey 2017). The news article implies that Rasoolan's in-laws had given up hope of her producing a child for the family and tying herself to them by becoming a mother. Rasoolan's natal family alleged that the attack on her would be an effective way of solving the problem of a presumably infertile daughter-in-law, despite the other legal possibilities available to her husband, Anees, as an Indian Muslim man, such as divorcing his wife or marrying another woman in addition to Rasoolan. The attack seems to have been produced by a breakdown in the fragile intimacies of the marital household and in the extended family's hopes for a child born of Rasoolan. I heard stories of the victimization of married women without children from others who knew of allegations about a neighbor or distant relatives. Harassment by in-laws emerged as a theme in these tales that circulated as "common knowledge," even without a known cast of individual actors. As the story about Rasoolan indicates, regardless of the status of infertility as a disease, and often regardless of the diagnosis by a medical or religious specialist, infertility can lead to significant human suffering and, in some extreme cases, death. Yet, in North Indian ideologies of motherhood, the emotional core of mothering is also a force that comes with peril, as it, too, is tied up with desire.

MOTHERLY AFFECTION: THE DANGERS OF DESIRE

"There is one door in the world that's never closed, and that door is a mother's affection [*ma ki mamta*] and a mother's love."
"*Duniya men ek darvaza aisa bhi hai jo kabhi band nahin hota hai aur vo darvaza hai ma ki mamta aur ma ka pyar.*"

—Farha Yasmeen, student at Karamat Hussain
Muslim Girls' Post-Graduate College, Lucknow (2004–05),
in the school magazine

In North Indian ideologies of motherhood, *ma ki mamta* (motherly affection) is a force of great significance. It can be seen as a source of unending and unchanging comfort for offspring but also as a sign of dangerous attachment to the things of the world. John Platts's *Dictionary of Urdu, Classical Hindi, and English* aligns with a religious renouncer's view of worldly relationships and defines the term *mamta* in an essentially negative light, emphasizing a misplaced sense of attachment. "*Mamta*: (Sanskrit origin) 'Egoism; the sense of "*meum*"; the interest, or affection, entertained for objects from the considering them as belonging to or connected with one's self; sense of ownership, or of self-interest; appropriation; selfishness; affection, attachment (to);—individuality; self-sufficiency; pride, arrogance; covetousness, avarice. *Mamta-yukt*: Filled with selfishness, self-interested, selfish; miserly;—an egotist, a selfish man, a miser'" (Platts 1977 [1884], 1067).

The affection of a mother, in the context of this understanding of the term *mamta*, acquires a different sheen than in the platitudes offered by Farha Yasmeen. A mother's affection can be dangerous and misguided, just as it can also be a source of reassurance for a child. In South Asia, grasping attachment to the things of this world is commonly cited across male-dominated religious traditions as a wrong-headed pursuit that should be overcome through religious devotion to attain higher spiritual realization. From the perspective of religious renunciation, *mamta*, and particularly the *mamta* of mothers, is a form of bondage to this world, a major stumbling block in the pursuit of release from the cycle of rebirth.

In families, however, *ma ki mamta* is a positive binding force, one that supports the development of children, the fulfillment of motherly aspirations, and the sentimental attachment that is supposed to promote family unity over the lifetime and inspire children to care for their parents as they age. In joint families, *ma ki mamta* needs to be moderated to promote the harmonious balance of relationships within the multigenerational household.

A mother's affectionate gaze can also unwittingly harm a child through the evil eye (*nazar lagna*, literally, "for the gaze to stick"), resulting in illness. The power and potential dangers of *ma ki mamta* echo throughout Indian popular culture. In the example of the 1987 Hindi film *Aulad* (cited below), motherly affection and love become dangerously disordered through the loss of a child and subsequent infertility, while ultimately offering a happy resolution to the crisis of an overabundance of *ma ki mamta*.

MOTHERLY AFFECTION: DESIRE
DIRECTED AND REDEEMED

In the 1987 Hindi film *Aulad* [*Progeny*] by director Vijay Sadanah and starring Jeetendra, Sridevi, Jayapradha, Saeed Jaffrey, Asrani, and Vinod Mehra, popular perceptions of the nature of motherly affection and child desire are explicitly explored and challenged through a tradition familiar to viewers of Hindi cinema, the idiom of Hindu mythology. The twists and turns of the plot align with viewer expectations of a Bollywood film. Many aspects of the storyline and characters' names align with the Hindu story of Lord Krishna, who was raised by a foster mother. Khare has discussed, in the context of his own fieldwork, the story of Lord Krishna as an example of the delineation of multiple types of mothers in the Hindu tradition, with emphasis on two main categories: the mother who gives birth to a child, and the mother who raises a child (Sadanah 1987).

> In Krishna's case, his birth-giving mother (Devaki) is overshadowed and equaled by Yashoda by following the dharma of being an actual mother even if she did not give birth to Krishna. In the popular conception, *mamta* of motherhood is present in every woman, and she can truly express it even if she is not a mother.

> These illustrations are another way to focus on the two basic components of motherhood: the act of giving birth (*apne peta se janama dena*) and rearing a child (*palana posana aur bara*

karana). . . . Normally, if it is admitted that a birth giving woman naturally (*svabhavatah*) develops an attachment toward her child, it is also argued that mother's true love (*ma ka saccha pyar*) is not limited to the birth-giving mother (*sacci ma*) alone. Intense *mamata* (attachment) of a foster mother like Yashoda is repeatedly described as the *dharma*-ordered ambience of true motherhood. (Khare 1982, 159–60)

The two major claimants to the role of mother in the 1987 film *Aulad* are patterned on these two mothers of Lord Krishna, Devki and Yashoda, a point that would not be lost on Indian viewers, whether watching in the 1980s or any time since then. Hindi films circulate for decades beyond their release dates through television screenings and repetition of their songs across radio, television, and the internet. The film deals with the question of which mother can be the true mother with great emotion but without conceding the possibility of multiple mothers for a single child. The film's main characters include Devki, who gives birth to the boy Kishen; her husband, Anand; and Yashoda, the woman who raises Kishen as her own son after a tragic train accident. In brief, Devki is lost and presumed dead after a train derailment when their newborn is scarcely one month old. The pregnant and injured Yashoda gives birth to a stillborn baby, and her husband is killed in the accident. Devki's husband, Anand, left alone with the infant boy Kishen, hears Yashoda's cries and pleads with the physician in charge to give Kishen to Yashoda to raise, while keeping Yashoda's stillbirth a secret, even from her. Expressing his inability to raise his infant son alone and unable to bear Yashoda's grief, Anand convinces the physician by saying, "She won't be able to live without a child. This is the only way to save her life. . . . Please don't delay, Doctor. A mother is in need of a child and a child is in need of a mother. . . . Doctor, this secret must remain secret for life. Yashoda's child is not dead, but alive. And I will forget that I ever had a child."[4]

Although Anand does indeed keep the secret from Yashoda, he cannot keep his promise to forget that he had a child. He develops a special affection for Kishen—whose name is a vernacular variant on Krishna—which others find strange. Scenes that reveal Kishen's "true" identity emphasize the importance of their connection. When Yashoda says that Kishen will follow the profession of his father, Anand misspeaks and says, "a businessman" (like himself), rather than a pilot, like Yashoda's late husband, and Kishen agrees that he wants to be a businessman. Throughout the film, Anand consistently affirms Yashoda's status as a mother, even to the point of denying his own wife the opportunity to reclaim their child when she mysteriously reappears four years later, after recovering from her injuries and amnesia thanks to the kind Kashmiri villagers who found her and took her in after the accident. Devki meets Kishen at Yashoda's place and senses some connection, which is dramatized by Kishen's affection for milk with Ovaltine, just like Anand. A voice echoes in Devki's head, signaling the importance of this similarity. Devki demands her child from the Hindu temple (*mandir*) where she and Anand had been married, asserting her right to her child, even though she had not been able to raise him (*parvarish*).

Still unaware that Yashoda has been raising the child she gave birth to, Devki meets both of them at the temple and tells Yashoda that she has great wealth (*daulat*) because she is a mother. Yashoda attempts to acknowledge Devki's pain, but she simultaneously denies her status as a mother, saying, "If God wills it, he'll fill your womb again." Shortly thereafter, however, Anand receives the diagnosis from a biomedical specialist that his wife will not be able to bear another child. The doctor notes that miracles sometimes happen, to which Anand responds, "Don't give us false comfort . . . I've understood that the joy of progeny (*aulad ka sukh*) is not in our destiny (*naseeb*)." It is important to note here that he uses the specific term *aulad*, rather than the more general *baccha* (child). The joy of which he speaks relates to a particular type of child—that is, progeny (*aulad*)—and suits the drama of his pronouncement.

As Devki learns the truth about Kishen's origins, the questions of who can truly be called his mother and the proper right to express *ma ki mamta* come into progressively sharper focus. In the temple to the goddess Durga where they had been married, Devki confronts Anand and learns that Kishen is the baby she gave birth to before her disappearance in the train accident, yet he claims that she has no right to him:

> **Devki:** I begged for a child in front of this mother, and she filled my womb. This Durga Ma is witness to my every moment.
>
> **Anand:** Kishen is our son.
>
> **Devki:** My son is alive. Mother, you protected the honor of my womb; I'm not a barren woman (*banjh*), I'm a mother.
>
> **Anand:** Listen, Devki, you aren't Kishen's mother . . .
>
> **Devki:** Why not? . . .
>
> **Anand:** That was one incident (*hadsa*), it was a moment . . . Kishen was the only one who could save Yashoda's life. I didn't know that the step I took out of humanity would one day become a problem, would become a question.
>
> **Devki:** I have the answer. Kishen is my son. I am his mother.
>
> **Anand:** Your tie (*rishta*) is only a relation of blood (*khun ka rishta*), the tie of mother (*ma ka rishta*) is Yashoda's. . . . Today she has nothing other than that child. Now Kishen is her only support (*sahara*).
>
> **Devki:** He's my future.
>
> **Anand:** A woman's other name is sacrifice (*qurbaani*). It's sacrifice (*balidaan*)!
>
> **Devki:** I'm not a woman, I'm a mother. I'm begging you! Don't come in the way of motherly affection (*mamta*). No one can halt the pull of blood (*khun ka taara*).

In great distress, Devki runs home to appeal to Lord Krishna, whose statue stands in their worship space there. Lord Krishna was the child who, in Hindu mythology, was raised not by the woman who gave birth to him but by Yashoda. Here the integral pairing of mother and child is apparent in Devki's agony over the continued denial of her status as a mother through the separation from Kishen. Her remonstrations before Lord Krishna point to the complexity of motherhood, the power of motherly attachment, and the dilemma presented by a case of too many claimants to an exclusive status of "mother."

> **Devki:** What sort of injustice is this? My child (*baccha*) is right in front of me and I'm wandering around looking for my child (*aulad*). If my child was to be given to Yashoda, then why did you give Kishen birth through my womb? Why did you make me a mother? Why did you give me the pain of affection (*mamta*)? Even being a mother, I couldn't call my own child my own. What kind of punishment is this? Oh God, what kind of test is this?

While Anand continues to give precedence to Yashoda's claim to the child as a mother based on her affection cultivated by raising the child and the absence of any other support or hope in life after the death of her husband, Devki asserts the priority of her claim to Kishen because of her embodied experience of pregnancy and birth. Yashoda, on learning about Kishen's origins, acknowledges this claim and demotes herself to the clearly inferior status of "the one who raised him" (*paalne wali*), even though she says that she "saw the light of her own motherly affection (*mamta*) in Kishen." The entire resolution of the film depends on resolving the question of whether the mother of Kishen is to be determined as biological, cultural, or perhaps biocultural—that is, combining both biological and cultural facets. As the conclusion approaches, momentum builds toward the recognition of Devki's biological claim, which Anand's uncle (mother's brother) asserts, saying, "Kishen's relation to us is one of blood (*khun*). . . . Kishen is our blood, he's the shining lamp of our family (*khandaan ka chiragh*). He'll only light up our home, no one else's!" Anand takes his argument to court and presents it eloquently, saying,

"Who is a mother? Is the only mother the one who gives birth? Isn't she a mother whose milk becomes blood and runs in the veins of the child? Isn't she a mother who has showered all of her affection (*mamta*) on a child? Isn't she a mother in whose heart is the pain of a child (*aulad ka dard*), whose every heartbeat is the call of a child? Your honor, I will say that if Yashoda Devi isn't Kishen's mother, then no woman in the world is the mother of her own child."

The judge sympathizes with Anand's sentiment but says that the law does not accept it: the law recognizes one cultural formulation of kinship—through birth and blood—over another, that of raising a child. Over Anand's objection, the court awards custody of the child to Anand and Devki as the biological parents. In this turn of events, Anand loses the argument by winning the right to the son he had never claimed as a biological father. However, the transfer of the child Kishen unravels the work of the court. He refuses to accept the new home as his own and runs away. Searching for Yashoda, he barely escapes death in a traffic accident, and this display of his affection for Yashoda changes Devki's mind about her claim on the boy. Finally, she relinquishes him to Yashoda, saying, "You are the only one who can give him a mother's affection (*mamta*)."[5]

The completion of this release seems to free Devki and set the world right. Devki faints, and, on awakening, she learns that, miraculously, she is pregnant and will again have the chance to become a mother. The implication is clear that the gods have smiled on her for her actions. By sacrificing her claim and making Yashoda an undisputed mother, she has redeemed herself to become a worthy mother in the most honored way. With great melodrama, the film sends the message that there are multiple ways to become a mother and that *ma ki mamta* can have multiple origins. Yet, social customs prioritizing motherhood through birth and blood are powerful, persuasive, and ensconced in law. In this case, the law does not have the final say, and eventually, the characters find the "right" one and only mother for this child and the "right" child (or promise of a child) for each mother. There is no suggestion of sharing mothering duties or claims to motherhood between Devki and Yashoda. Blood and birth do not win the day, and the film suggests that this outcome puts the world back in order. Both Devki's and Yashoda's hunger, their desire for children expressed through *ma ki mamta*, is satisfied, enabling them to live, both in the sense of bodily existence and as respectable members of society.

In *Aulad*, the importance of becoming a mother is paramount; however, motherly status and recognition unravel in ways that strain the women to their limits. A variety of claims to motherly affection through the womb, blood, milk, and the act of raising a child parse out what in most women's experiences become a unified bundle of ties that secure their rights in their child but may still not protect them from loss in the face of marital dissolution or their child's (and especially son's) changing priorities.

POPULAR WISDOM ABOUT BECOMING MOTHERS IN LUCKNOW

Women across the social spectrum and of diverse religious and class backgrounds in Lucknow stressed to me the importance of becoming mothers (*ma banna*), no matter what else women might do in life. These included women who had pursued other goals in life besides motherhood and had careers as teachers, writers, and social activists. Many of them, whether or not they worked outside their homes, expressed that women who worked outside their homes were better equipped to deal with infertility problems. They opined that these women would not be as seriously afflicted by not becoming mothers because they had other ways to spend their time and because the desires of other family members would not occupy their attention to such a great extent. In my interviews in infertility clinics, doctors and women seeking treatment discussed the stakes of infertility problems for women who worked outside their homes and women who worked only within their homes. They agreed that women working outside the home had more leverage to make excuses about why they had not yet become mothers and that they could pass time in ways other than caring for children. Women who were dealing with the effects of infertility often shared these sentiments with women of other reproductive profiles, both professionals and those whose primary tasks involved managing their own households. I found that women in Lucknow framed the importance of becoming mothers within the complex web of relationships among members of the extended family, which can be intricate and have significant consequences for women's lives in the *sasural* (in-laws' home, the "marigold" of chapter 1). The importance of becoming a mother could be understood as a particular refraction of the desire for children, and especially for *aulad*. The arrival of progeny signals the start of new social relationships. Several teachers at a Muslim women's college in the city were quite discriminating in observing that the effects of infertility could vary significantly depending on whether the couple suffering from infertility lived in, for example, large cities—"metros," such as Delhi, Calcutta/Kolkata, Bombay/Mumbai, Madras/Chennai, and Bangalore/Bengaluru—or small towns.

For married couples, the implications of not becoming parents could relate not only to the attitudes of family members but also to job opportunities available—although most agreed that the stigma of infertility is not bound by economic status—and the likelihood that infertile couples lived in joint versus nuclear families. In joint families, as my interlocutors told it, couples feel greater pressure to "oblige" their family members with a child. Again, the significant locus of desire is not only with husbands or wives but also with their extended family members, especially husbands' mothers. The unique centrality of "becoming a mother" might be about experiencing pregnancy and giving

birth, but the physical experiences were only one part of motherhood, and not less important than the matrix of status and relationships that becoming a mother created, with all its fragility
and shifting potential.

I noted my own surprise at the number of women who talked
about the differences that could arise in women's experiences of
dealing with infertility based on class, education, place of residence, and so on but who would disavow any suggestion that
women's religious identity would make any difference in their experiences. On this point, most women argued that the stigma of
childlessness goes beyond religious background and that women
will go to any length to get children. Further, most agreed that
women would not abide by boundaries imposed by religion in
seeking a solution for their problem, and that all women were
ultimately united in this common experience of suffering. They
drew examples from stories, films, mythology, and history to
speak about the possible ways of dealing with childlessness. Muslim women were more willing to entertain the possibility of living
without children than women from other religious backgrounds,
and they often referred to Islamic texts.[6] Although they rarely
mentioned specific Quranic quotations, Muslim women often
noted that the Quran says that not everyone will be given children and that this was a basis for comfort in the face of reproductive difficulties.

The Mughal emperor Akbar (ruled 1556–1605, known as a great
proponent of religious tolerance) was reputed to have fertility
problems, and stories about Akbar have made sites related to
his life, especially the shrine (*mazaar*) of Sufi saint Salim Chishti at Fatepur Sikri, near the Taj Mahal (in Agra, western Uttar
Pradesh), a focus of some women's fertility pilgrimages. One of
my closest friends and interlocutors during my fieldwork was a
young woman from a Sunni Muslim background, a *sayyid* (member of a high-status Muslim group) who lived in the old city. She
was highly educated and not yet married. She told me about mem-

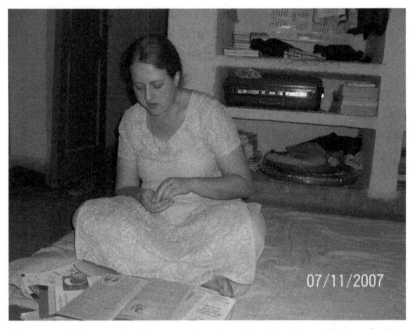

07/11/2007

Figure 2.1. At home in Lucknow, evaluating educational pamphlets and other written materials gathered in the field. The embroidery on this *shalwar kameez* is done in typical midrange Lucknowi *chikan*-style on thin cotton fabric. (Photo by author.)

bers of her extended family who were involved in healing through the use of *taaviz,* amulets with religious verses or numerological formulas inscribed or tucked inside them on slips of paper. After we had known each other for some time, she suggested that I speak with one of her relatives on the phone about my research, though she hesitated to introduce me to him in person. She grew up in a family that observed many conservative social traditions but that had acquiesced to her wish to pursue advanced studies, to work, and to travel locally on her own without observing purdah through covering or concealment in a closed vehicle. Based on these varied interactions and experiences, she argued that childlessness could be interpreted as a gift from God that should be accepted, but she also reflected that people would generally feel the lack of a child in their lives if this were to happen to them.

Among women in my fieldwork who were seeking infertility treatment in biomedical clinics, there were significant differences of opinion about the practice of exercising such strategies in the pursuit of motherhood. Some women vehemently argued that women in their situation were so desperate that any child would be better than no child at all, and that it did not matter whether the child was male or female. Others stated that they would like to have a male child. In the clinical context, other questions could arise, such as whether or not it would be acceptable to try for pregnancy using donor sperm if the male partner was found to have fertility problems. Some women—some couples, since both had to sign permission for the procedure—saw this as an acceptable method of pursuing motherhood. Yet, the head nurse in the unit told me that there were couples who refused this line of treatment. Their pragmatics would not go so far as to accommodate the possibility of creating a parent-child relationship through donated sperm. Anxieties about using donor sperm often revolved around issues of "blood" and how such children would "fit" with their parents and within the household, so the concerns were about relationships with parents, but also with larger kin networks.

DESTABILIZING IDEOLOGIES OF MOTHERHOOD: INDIAN AND CROSS-CULTURAL PERSPECTIVES

Feminist scholars have critiqued motherhood in a plethora of ways that have emphasized patriarchy, control of female sexuality, and the use and abuse of female bodies and labor in reproductive tasks, among others (Ragoné and Twine 2000; Rothman 1990). Motherhood has been described in many cultures as the attainment of full status as an adult and as a woman, a crucial part of the life course that makes infertility a crushing blow to a woman's social status. However, feminist scholars have also examined the contingencies of motherhood and how motherhood may be better understood not as a once-and-for-all achievement but as a stage in a process, one that may be undone or the benefits of which may in some ways be fleeting. Recent scholarship in the anthropology of reproduction has demonstrated the many ways that motherhood as a construct can be destabilized by analyzing changing patterns of relationships over a lifetime and through examination of the impact of various reproductive woes on the definition of a mother. Cross-cultural examples provide ample evidence for changes in the importance of women's identities as mothers over time, and for the ways that people who give birth become and un-become mothers (Johnson-Hanks 2006). Reproduction is at best a fragile process, and the point at which reproduction can be said to be successful varies depending on cultural specificities.

Rayna Rapp (1999) and Linda Layne (2003) have both given powerful accounts of the outer boundaries of motherhood and the heartache that can accompany the loss of a wanted pregnancy, and with it, the full claim to being a mother. In Rapp's case, most women "chose" the loss of their baby-to-be because of a positive diagnosis of fetal abnormalities, the most common of which was Down's syndrome. The great majority of the New York women in the study expressed their helplessness in the face of the situation to make any other decision, and Rapp noted that women without other living children suffered greatly at the loss of their potential child, while women with other children recovered more quickly. One major factor here is certainly the loss of a potential identity as a mother—and that, too, of an idealized child—that these women had anticipated as an outcome of their pregnancies until receiving the diagnosis (Rapp 1999, 246).

Layne's work on pregnancy loss highlights the total lack of choice experienced by American women who lost pregnancies spontaneously; that is, they suffered what is commonly referred to as a miscarriage or, in some cases, a stillbirth. For those who sought support through groups, such as the one whose newsletter serves as a major source of the book's data, pregnancy loss was a threat to their personhood, their status as parents, and especially to their status as parents to a particular child-to-be who, according to friends and family, never quite was. Layne's moving material culture analysis demonstrates how parents-to-be who have experienced pregnancy loss or stillbirth attempt to establish the reality of their lost child-to-be, and sometimes to establish their own status as parents, through the accumulation of such simulacra as baby shoes, sonogram images, and documents such as the "Recognition of Life" certificate, which stand in for a birth certificate and other material items that a surviving baby would acquire (2003, 137). Both Rapp and Layne highlight the tenuous relationship between procreation and the social recognition of mothers, depending on the outcome of pregnancy, and American ambiguities about when mothers can legitimately claim that status.[7]

The vagaries of biological reproduction are far from the only relevant doubts in making mothers or in attaining a culturally recognized state of motherhood. Jennifer Johnson-Hanks has argued that, in Cameroon, some women—especially very young women—are able to give birth, but they avoid the status of motherhood and preserve for themselves the chance of becoming "honorable" mothers later in life. An example of this is a young mother relinquishing a child to the biological father's family and returning to school (Johnson-Hanks 2002, 878). Here the biological fact of having given birth to a child need not determine the young woman's identity nor radically change her life course, and she can potentially sidestep or postpone the obligations of being a mother, depending on how she navigates this "vital conjuncture" (Johnson-Hanks 2002, 2006).

Johnson-Hanks points to one constellation of culturally sanctioned moves that render biology irrelevant at the potential inception of motherhood. Other potential examples include surrendering a newborn for adoption, abandoning an infant, or entering into a surrogacy contract, depending on the cultural context. Sarah Lamb (2000) destabilized motherhood at the end of life, in the context of relationships between mothers and sons in the Eastern Indian state of West Bengal. The elderly village women with whom Lamb conducted her fieldwork argued that, due to the effects of modernization on employment, lifestyles, and gender relations, motherhood is a status of only passing importance. They portrayed mothers as selfless givers who pour out their labor and sacrifice their very bodies for the sake of their children, especially their sons, but their efforts are never returned in measure. However, the blame for this neglect tends to fall on their sons' wives, who are anyway suspect outsiders, and who are anxious to look after the needs of their own children at the expense of their husband's parents (2000, 75–78). In both the examples from Cameroon and West Bengal, motherhood as a social status can be seen to ebb and flow over a lifetime; it is not coterminous with pregnancy or birth. The questions of who is a mother when, and how much it matters are of great consequence cross-culturally and can stimulate much debate. For example, do the communities around women who have given birth to children that did not survive still consider them to be mothers? How might the answer to that question matter for the conditions of their lives going forward?

In my fieldwork, women spoke not about the state of motherhood but about *becoming* mothers (*ma banna*).[8] The expression includes the transformation of status and the process involved, but it does not attribute agency in bringing about the transformation. A similar expression might be used for making *rotis*, the round wheat flatbread that accompanies most meals in Uttar Pradesh. To say *roti banni hai* means that the rotis need to be made but does not specify who will make them. That would require a different verb, *banāna*. The extra syllable allows for agency, and it is the verb that people usually use when they ask, for example, "When will you make me an auntie?" For women seeking help from biomedical clinics, the ideal way to become a mother was certainly through the course of their own pregnancy, even though they might need to enlist the help of doctors, other medical professionals, and possibly even gamete donors. In their desperation to become mothers, women in those spaces idealized both the status of mothers and the potential effects that children would have on their lives and their relationships. This position finds a great deal of support in popular literature and among women I met beyond clinics, but it is certainly not without its critics in India.

Remembering her experiences of motherhood, Nabaneeta Dev Sen, a scholar and former wife of economist Amartya Sen, recalls her feelings at hearing the fetus's heartbeat in her first pregnancy, writing,

> I was genuinely happy, but at the same time I suddenly felt suffocated and trapped. I felt my freedom as a person was lost forever. . . . Once a mother, forever a mother. You are duty-bound for all time. You can never be a free woman. I felt trepidations. . . . Was I good enough to be a mother? Kind enough? Honest enough? Could I make sacrifices? A mother must be all of these. No. I was not fit for the role of motherhood. . . . Surely not me. . . . Motherhood was too glorious a role to be played properly by me. (Sen 2006, 119)

Nabaneeta Dev Sen's portrayal of motherhood as unfreedom provides an interesting counterpoint to Amartya Sen's more well-known critiques of the idea of freedom (1999). This account appears in an English-language collection of writings about mothers and motherhood by South Asian women, most of them highly educated and successful scholars and writers. The title, *Janani*, is evocative in that the term comes from the Sanskrit lexicon of Hindi, meaning "mother" in the very specific biological sense of a birthing woman. Sen emphasizes well-worn constructions of motherhood in South Asia, including the eternity of motherhood, the necessity of sacrificing for the good of one's children, and the imperative to be an ideal model of the "mother." Sen describes how her life experiences, including the breakup of her marriage, challenged her vision of motherhood and of herself as a mother.

In the same collection, Shashi Deshpande writes about discovering how the ideals about motherhood she learned from her upbringing—that a mother sacrifices all for her children, and that a woman is a refuge for her children—proved to be quite different from the realities she saw as an adult, before and after becoming a mother herself (2006, 131–32). She grew into bitter realizations about mothers, that "they can stifle their children's desires, that mothers who say they want nothing for themselves, try to get things through their children, a mother's sacrifice can become a rope to tether her children to herself, that it can be used as a weapon in the never-ending mother-child warfare" (2006, 132).

Deepa Gahlot, who identifies herself as a childfree adult woman beyond the age of thirty-four, derides her friends for suggesting that she needs to adopt a child so that she can become an adult. First, she takes issue with the need to attain adult status, and second, she describes motherhood as "lifelong bondage" to which she would never submit herself (2006, 138–39). Sen's and Deshpande's narratives demonstrate the differences between the kinds of advice about and representations of motherhood they knew growing up and the realities they saw as they became mothers themselves and witnessed mothering by others. Gahlot's story travels far afield from mainstream South Asian representations of mothers, such as Farha Yasmeen's Urdu platitudes about mothers[9] and the glorification of mothers and motherhood in *Aulad*, and challenges women (and people of all genders, for that matter) to justify the need for children, beyond sustaining the species.

In her study of North Indian infertility clinics in the late 1990s, Anjali Widge found that some women were less interested in the pursuit of a child than in the pursuit of their own self-dignity, which they sought to secure through a child. One of the women she interviewed, a forty-year-old Punjabi Hindu housewife, who had been seeking infertility treatment for ten years, put it this way: "My mother-in-law called me a eunuch, blamed and threatened me, said that I will be thrown out. Not that I wanted my own child so badly . . . especially when I got to know that it is going to be with a donor's sperm . . . but I wanted to prove that I am a woman" (2005, 229).

This woman's childless state caused her to suffer not only from missing motherhood but also from aspersions cast on her identity as a complete woman. The reference to being a eunuch can imply that one is neither fully male nor female but is similar to those known as *hijras* or *kinnar*, identified around the world as "third sex" or "third gender" people of India (Reddy 2005; Nanda 1990). Here, the implications of the mother-in-law's threats are even more poignant, since doctors must have identified male-factor infertility as at least one source of the woman's inability to produce children. Romantic conceptions of motherhood are prevalent in South Asian culture in many forms, including the various representations of mother goddesses and popular Islamic valorizations of motherhood—such as the famous saying "Heaven lies at the feet of the mother."

Changing gender roles and employment opportunities are leading some women to question motherhood's place in comparison to upward mobility on their own. Some elite Indian women are questioning the value of becoming mothers, not only because they can find financial support elsewhere and need not depend on the prospects of sons but also because emotional support and intimacy from children as comfort in old age are far from guaranteed. Recent economic transformations support such critiques, particularly for already advantaged Indians who have been in a position to benefit most from the liberalization reforms of the 1990s. Connection to a child through genetics, blood, gestation, milk, or other culturally relevant substances does not guarantee that selfless affection will develop between mother and child. Neither does the absence of such ties preclude the development of affection, as part of a long process of forging emotional relationships between mother and child.

Critics of the idea of universal, automatic mother love have often pointed to the ways that some mothers seem to deliberately withhold their affection and attachment toward their children for some time after their birth. This reservation has been linked to conditions of high infant mortality and to the slow attribution of personhood to children through institutions such as the naming of the child or the sharing of food and bodily fluids (Conklin and Morgan 1996, 658). Rapp's work on amniocentesis and selective abortion based on the results of amniocentesis, especially in the diagnosis of disorders such as Down's syndrome, and Janelle Taylor's (2008) work on the use of ultrasound for "bonding" during pregnancy in the contemporary United States demonstrate that the "pragmatics of motherhood" and "bonding" can be fostered long before birth through the use of technologies intended to reveal the nature of the fetus. The ethical implications of these technologies are many and varied, particularly since the same technologies are deployed to different ends, depending on the acceptability of particular birth outcomes. For example, some people may consider the diagnosis of a chromosomal abnormality to be legal, ethical, and/or pragmatic grounds for terminating a pregnancy; in other cases within the United States and around the world, the sex of the fetus may be the more compelling grounds for acceptance or rejection of burgeoning parenthood. This can be observed, for example, in the large-scale abortion of female fetuses through the use of ultrasound and other tests for determining fetal sex in places such as China and India and in global diasporic populations. In India, this illegal practice is known as "foeticide" (feticide), is subject to a variety of feminist critiques in a place where abortion rights in general are largely undisputed, and is most prevalent in the wealthiest northern states (Visaria 2007, 64–65).

The solutions physicians offered to overcome or circumvent infertility problems had great potential to come into conflict with the values women articulated to me about creating families. Ideologies about becoming mothers, directing child desire, and maintaining hope certainly informed the actions of women suffering from reproductive disruption in Lucknow during the time of my research. Religious identity and access to financial resources also played significant roles in the expanding or limiting options that women could pursue in hopes of successful reproduction. Among women seeking children in Lucknow, I did not hear expressed desires to be "a free woman"—quite the contrary, women sought to cultivate and strengthen bonds through children. One day, in the waiting room of a large government infertility clinic, a particularly eager group of women were waiting for the doctor to arrive so that they could begin their exams and find out which procedures would be performed that day. When I told them about my project, they all agreed to take part and promptly launched into a discussion about society and infertility that I found myself nearly powerless to direct. I enjoyed the flow of it but feared that the women's voices would infuriate the medical staff in the next room. Several agreed that women suffer from problems and worries (*pareshaani*) regardless of whether or not they have children. Amid this discussion, a particularly outspoken Sikh woman brought others to agreement by arguing forcefully, "Whatever happens, the one who has nobody . . . to become a mother is the most important [biggest] job. That poor lady . . . outsiders say. The one who doesn't have any [children] learns what their importance (*ahamiyat*) is."[10]

Yet, the birth of children in and of itself does not guarantee the joy or relief promised by the prospect of *aulad*. Some reasons relate to local ways of understanding the nature of *aulad* in terms of the sex of children or their biological relationship with their families, for example, but also to the very real possibility that children may not survive. As the contemporary practice of

gestational surrogacy in India and around the world demonstrates, gestating a pregnancy and giving birth to a child does not
automatically grant women the status of being a mother. Conception, pregnancy, and birth do not in and of themselves naturally
make mothers, and Indian tradition lends some support to the
idea of differentiating mothering roles between birthing and raising a child. Specialists who facilitate surrogacy take advantage of
these ideas as well as of genetic reckonings of kinship to convince
prospective surrogates (and their partners) that the children
born from their wombs under surrogacy arrangements do not
belong to them. However, portrayals of mothering as in the stories of Krishna and the characters in the film *Aulad* do offer the
possibility of claims to rights in a child beyond those produced
through DNA swabs or the evidence of birth, even as the labors
of pregnancy and birth disappear from view. Although genetic
reckoning of motherhood excludes some women who give birth
from the status of motherhood, some versions of "tradition" lend
credence to the idea that women can become mothers without
giving birth, by participating in raising children. As in many parts
of the world, the terrain of mothering is hotly contested ground
in contemporary India, yet its contours emerge in the particular landscape of ideals about gender and building families. The
importance of these ideals for women's lives begins even before
marriage through control of women's education, movement, and
sexual expression, and it has significant implications for their
lives throughout and beyond the span of their reproductive careers, wherever those journeys may lead them.

NOTES

1. A pseudonym.
2. Dr. Kapoor, patient information session, July 4, 2005.
3. Platts's *Dictionary of Urdu, Classical Hindi, and English* glosses the
word *yateem* as "a fatherless child, an orphan; a pupil, ward" (Platts [1884]
1977). In this context, the emphasis is clearly on the absence of a mother.

4. The English translations throughout are mine.

5. In Hindi: Devki: "Mamta tum hi de sakti ho" (*Aulad*: 2:43).

6. For example, stories such as that of Mary, Zakariya, and Ishba, from the Quran:

> "As with the story of Ibrahim (peace be upon him) we have the example of a husband who remains with his barren wife. She is not shunned, shammed [*sic*], divorced, or looked down upon as an incomplete woman as many men and cultures do to women. This is a lesson that all of our ummah must learn, as Allah says 'He leaves barren whom He wills' (42: 50)." Accessed June 14, 2021. http://www.angelfire.com/la/IslamicView/Quran1.html.

7. Points at which the status of motherhood can be lost are also certainly up for debate in the American context, as demonstrated by, for example, legal battles over adoption cases and famous cases involving custody battles with surrogates hired to bear children, sometimes using their own ova, and sometimes by gestating an embryo created by an intending couple (Dolgin 1997).

8. The most commonly used phrase in Urdu for motherhood refers to being or becoming a mother (*ma ka hona* or *ma banna*); there is no equivalent term for motherhood in common usage as there is for fatherhood (*abuiyyat*).

9. Her pithy sayings from the Karamat Hussain College magazine appear earlier in this chapter. One more radiant example of the idealization of mothers in her sayings: *"Jis ghar men talim yafta aur nek dil ma ho to vo ghar tehzeeb o insaniyat ki university hai."* ("The house in which an educated and pure-hearted mother dwells is a university of refinement and humanity.")

10. Quote from a woman seeking infertility treatment in a Lucknow hospital, fieldnotes November 2007.

THREE

CLINICAL DREAMS

Measuring Hope

We are without support . . . when you don't have someone of your own, no one else comes to take their place.

—Mamta, seeking infertility treatment, 2007

AS I LOOK BACK ON my notes from the early days of my field-work in Lucknow, I am reminded of all the time I spent visiting the offices of gynecologists, or "lady doctors," in local parlance, at small private practices. Many times, a friend or acquaintance suggested that I visit a doctor or clinic. My mother-in-law even took me to meet the doctor who oversaw her care and my husband's birth nearly thirty-five years earlier. She was still practicing, and my mother-in-law found her clinic easily. I went to clinics in many different parts of the city during the doctors' posted times to see patients, the only time the doctor's presence in the clinic could be reasonably well-assured. At other times of the day, the physician might be resting, visiting other patients, practicing at another facility, performing an operation, or going about the mundane details of daily life. In the early days of 2005 and 2006, I spent many hours waiting—waiting for doctors to arrive and waiting for a moment when they might speak with me. In the meantime, I took in the scenes of the waiting rooms full of women and the people who accompanied them. At these clinics, pregnant women, children, husbands, and other friends or relatives crowded into the small waiting rooms. Ceiling fans cooled the nicer rooms but were still inadequate to provide relief from the heat for most of the year. Women with all kinds of concerns about their reproductive health could visit these clinics. They mingled in the waiting room and often saw the physician in groups of two or three. There was no guarantee of privacy here— more likely the guarantee of no privacy. Some visitors milled around outside while waiting for their turns. For women seeking solutions to infertility problems, a place like this, often situated near a market or within a residential area, since physicians often set up clinical spaces within their own homes, might be their first stop. Women I interviewed in larger clinics often narrated their journeys from one doctor to another, in their own towns and in different parts of Lucknow, before they reached more specialized infertility centers. My notes from the time I spent seeking clinics where I could observe how infertility was handled through clinical treatment reflect the richness and confusion of these small clinics.

Memories of past abuses, including, for example, a history of forced sterilizations and ongoing anxieties about reproduction across caste and religious categories that healthcare providers and patients both carry into hospitals, haunt the provision of care for reproductive health and fertility services in India. The ethnographic work I have done on infertility treatment in small gynecological clinics and in large hospitals over the last decade dissuades me from making overarching proclamations about the ethos of particular institutions. However, that has not stopped my interlocutors from sharing their perceptions about what individual hospitals were like, especially how they treated patients from diverse backgrounds. Intense treatment encounters in infertility units in hospitals give some patients hope—their presence signals that they are worthy of care and that technology may help them fulfill their reproductive aspirations. However, many of my interlocutors outside of hospitals argued that stereotypes about some prospective patients as "bad" patients and hyperfertile, antimodern people kept them from using public services. For those who entered hospitals as patients, these spaces are both familiar and strange—familiar in the power differentials between medical staff and patients, strange in their jargon and procedures. Care may be given, withheld, recognized, misrecognized, hidden, or discarded in multiple ways in clinical spaces as patients navigate their affective needs between home and hospital in search of children. These small and large actions show how the discourses of clinical staff and the people who seek their help are integral to coproducing science and modernity (Jasanoff 2004) in hospitals, in ways that are rooted in fractures of religion, caste, class, and gender in India. Here, I approach quests for children in Lucknow through the institutions most recognizable in Western and contemporary analyses of infertility—gynecologists' offices and biomedical infertility clinics.

Medical doctors, including general gynecologists and specialists in infertility treatment in government and private practice, whom I interviewed during my research in Lucknow tended to express broad views about the appropriate ways of resolving infertility. These doctors were nearly exclusively female. Most people in India see gynecology as an appropriate specialization for women entering medicine, and female patients generally feel more comfortable with exams conducted by female doctors. There were relatively fewer specialists who focused on male-factor infertility, although occasionally urologists or andrologists were available for consultation. They were not, however, directly part of the infertility units I visited, and I did not have the opportunity to interview them. I found gynecologists to be quite busy and often brusque, although they were less so in conversations with me than when examining patients. Most had a long line of patients waiting to be seen in a relatively short period.

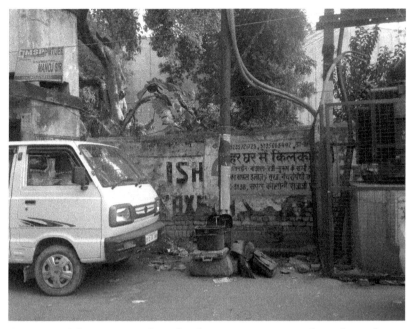

Figure 3.1. Advertisement for infertility treatment painted on a boundary wall near the Lucknow Zoo. In Hindi, sandwiched between two electricity poles with some of the text obscured, the ad promises successful treatment of childlessness/sterility due to male and female factors through naturopathy and provides an address for the clinic and mobile phone numbers for inquiries. (Photo by author.)

Dr. Ahmed

One of the first physicians I met was an elderly Muslim woman, Dr. Sadiya Ahmed,[1] who had been a practicing "lady doctor" for decades in her clinic just off a congested, dusty market near the military cantonment. Women could go out to the market and also visit the doctor, although they might need to explain the long absence from home that a visit to Dr. Ahmed could mean. I had been told that her patients came from the surrounding area. Many arrived on foot and were fully clad in long black burqas (burqā) that covered their forms and concealed all but the most advanced pregnancies. In this state of cover, and even for women wearing other common forms of loose Indian dress, it would have been difficult, if not impossible, to distinguish a woman suffering from infertility from one seeking birth control or care for all but the most advanced pregnancies, ensuring greater privacy for them and more challenges for anyone seeking to direct or talk with them based on their particular concern. During our first visit together, Dr. Ahmed gave me advice about studying infertility and potential solutions to infertility, based on her experience treating and advising the patients who visited her. She displayed a particular kind of local expertise bolstered by her biomedical credentials and her Urdu speech, which invoked old Lucknow in its rhythm and in the sounds carried over from its Persian and Arabic connections. Over time, I came to recognize the commanding presence and extreme conviction and confidence she displayed in her bearing and speech as a common trait among "lady doctors." When we met for a second time, I wrote in my fieldnotes that

> I mentioned that I would be interested in talking with some patients being treated for infertility. She seemed very willing to let me do this, but a little perplexed about how exactly to manage it, since infertility patients can turn up any time. How would I be able to set any schedule to see them? I mentioned that I could bring some information about my study and contact information and they said that I could do that if I felt it would be appropriate. They didn't see any need for it. So, I need to figure out a way to see these patients without spending all day every day sitting in the clinic waiting for a case to turn up.

I did not do further research at her clinic, but she gave me clues and referrals that got me thinking about the local dynamics of infertility treatment and the larger context of infertility experiences in Lucknow.

Dr. Godrej

Another Lucknow clinic I visited at the beginning of my work was a center affiliated with an international family-planning organization. Larger than Dr. Ahmed's clinic and with more staff members, this clinic was just off a wide road in an upscale residential area not far from Lucknow University. It was not the kind of place women were likely to stumble into by accident or be able to easily explain to neighbors or acquaintances who might spot them there. However, the relative isolation of this clinic made accidental discovery somewhat unlikely compared to Dr. Ahmed's office. While waiting for the doctor in charge, I noticed charts hanging on the wall, which listed statistics about procedures performed in the previous year: nearly 2,000 sterilizations (1 male), almost 400 infertility checkups (6 conceived), and over 8,000 total patients seen.[2] Dr. Bita Godrej held responsibility for this clinic, and she talked matter-of-factly with me about how her experiences running the clinic and visiting rural areas around Lucknow during her five years there had influenced how she saw infertility and related issues. Her stridency comes through in the detailed notes I took after the interview but in a way that now seems muted by my efforts to get down just what she said, and not to react. Unlike most of the women I spoke with in clinics, many doctors chose to converse in English, Dr. Godrej among them.

> Dr. Godrej said that the infertility services they provided are also available at government hospitals. However, many people find that the government facilities are not very user-friendly. One big difference between this clinic and the other facilities is that this one provides a lot of counseling, and counsels every patient (even husband and wife) separately.... She says that patients who come for infertility treatment come entirely through word of mouth. She also said that patients often come here last—after they have consulted "quacks" and spent a lot of money. People come from many places in U.P., including Faizabad, Gorakhpur, and Sitapur. While the clinic provides counseling, it does not give patient literature. Dr. Godrej says that most of the patients are illiterate. Dr. Godrej said that husbands often don't want their wives to know if they have fertility problems because of male "ego." Yet infertility is always blamed on the woman.

The clinic performs abortions only up to the 12th week of pregnancy. Sometimes people with more advanced pregnancies come in asking for abortions. In many cases, these are patients who have found out that the fetus is female and want to abort. They chase these people away. Dr. Godrej comments that she visits a particular village every Saturday and that, seeing the lives of women there, she wonders whether female feticide [sex-selective abortion] is really wrong.

Dr. Godrej says that social structure plays a big role in infertility. Mothers-in-law don't want to admit that something could be wrong with their sons. Plus, they often have a superiority complex about reproduction because they have produced sons. Dr. Godrej says that education is key, but that the attitude of the childbearing woman is only part of the picture, and that the roles of the mother-in-law and husband are also crucial.

Dr. Godrej expressed a definite bias toward biomedical approaches and criticized the "quacks" and others who profit from infertility patients. She says that infertility is not a problem for the government, but that, for couples facing childlessness, it's a very big social problem.

Dr. Godrej immediately took the issue of infertility as an expression of the hierarchies within a woman's marital household, whereby in-laws tend to blame the woman and avoid any doubt that their son could be the source of infertility, mirroring the themes expressed by Dr. Kapoor in her patient-education sessions. She emphasized the mother-in-law's role of harassing a woman without children, saying that they often have a superiority complex toward their daughter-in-law because they themselves had been successful in producing a son (thus enabling them to become mothers-in-law; that is, *saases*, with *bahus*, daughters-in-law). This doctor, who lived in New Delhi for many years before moving to Lucknow, went so far as to say that, seeing the lives of women in Uttar Pradesh and especially in the village that she visited regularly on weekends, she wondered whether the practice of selective abortion of female fetuses was really wrong. She mused that women's lives were hard and that men were needed to earn a living in villages, so maybe it would be better if there were more men than women in villages. Still, the practice has generated sufficient political will that identifying a fetus's sex through means such as ultrasound is banned, initially in 1994, with revisions in 2002.[3] Few doctors were able or willing to take the time during their interactions with women in clinics to provide such thoughtful analysis of these issues, and few clinics employed a professional counselor to advise people seeking treatment.

Aside from Dr. Kapoor's patient-education meetings conducted in her private clinic, I heard of few cases of a doctor actually sitting down with patients in a forum like the one Dr. Kapoor arranged to explain the course of infertility treatment, the possible alternatives, and the implications of treatment in social and financial terms. For most patients, however, information was communicated on a spottier need-to-know basis. For example, doctors or nurses explained which medicines needed to be taken and how often, writing down their prescriptions on a sheet of paper with lines and circles to indicate how many times a day the medicine should be taken. They explained which tests would need to be done and where, but very rarely would women or their companions receive an explanation of why. This type of doctor-patient interaction exists across medical specialties in South Asia (and beyond), where doctors keep busy schedules and significant power differentials between doctor and patient inhibit patients from extensive questioning about the course of treatment.

Other gynecologists in Lucknow expressed perspectives similar to Dr. Kapoor's to me, such as a willingness to suggest adoption to people consulting them for infertility problems, especially adopting a child from outside of one's own extended family through official channels such as adoption agencies. Many people suffering from infertility suggested the option of raising the child of a family member as one way of relieving their childlessness, but doctors generally counseled against this, not as a way of increasing their revenue for infertility treatment but to avert the pain caused by the biological parents interfering in the child's upbringing. Medical doctors, who specialized in facilitating normative biological parenthood—or some approximation of that ideal—did not categorically promote the production of progeny and the forging of parent-child relationships through the assisted reproductive techniques (ARTs) they could provide. However, suggestions about other courses of action, in most cases, went only as far as verbal advice, not as far as actual structured counseling or concrete information about how to pursue adoption.

Only a few of the several private infertility clinics in Lucknow enjoy good reputations among people I spoke with during my fieldwork, and women mentioned the same places to me again and again, regardless of whether they had personally been involved in infertility treatment. Government (public) hospitals charge much lower fees for consultation with physicians and for medical tests than private institutions, but patients with sufficient means often avoid these facilities because of their reputations for administrative hassles and poor treatment by the staff. Doctors have been known by patients to use their position in government institutions to build their professional reputations, then open private medical practice or associated laboratory facilities. This enables them not only to reap the financial benefits of private practice that are available to well-known and well-reputed doctors who can develop a following through years of public practice and sometimes through media exposure but also to attain a degree of autonomy that remains impossible in the public sector. It made sense for me to examine infertility treatment in government hospitals because their care is theoretically open to all people at relatively lower fees and because their treatment regimen depends on government mandates for spending. "Family planning" has been prevalent in government facilities for decades, but in common usage and mostly in practice it has meant only the provision of birth control. Advanced infertility treatment in government facilities is still only available in a limited number of hospitals. It is not surprising, then, that women traveled long distances to Lucknow, the state capital, to pursue treatment.

LUCKNOW INFERTILITY CLINICS: CENTERS FOR CREATING SECRETLY "MODERN" LIVES

Infertility as a medical condition has complex origins, not all of which can be thoroughly diagnosed and treated by biomedicine. Infertility is nothing new in the world, and neither is the existence of ritual, kinship, and/or healing arts interventions to remedy the sense of reproductive failure that often accompanies infertility. Cultural context is key to making sense of infertility. Infertility may be defined in particular cultural contexts as the inability to conceive or to produce a living child, but it may also be defined as the inability to produce as many children as one desires or to produce the sex of children one desires. Similarly, understanding child desire also requires attention to the diverse ways people in particular cultural contexts dream about children—the number and sex of those children, their complexions, their abilities, and their origins. Just as diversity abounds in terms of how infertility and the desire for children are understood as problems, the same is true of strategies for dealing with infertility to obtain wanted children. I set out to understand women's experiences of infertility and those results as they sought children they could define and claim within their families and society as their "own."

The introduction and expansion of infertility treatment services in government facilities is part of a shift in priorities in reproductive health planning following the United Nations 1994 International Conference on Population and Development in Cairo (Visaria et al. 1999). The government of India dropped the use of numerical targets for people accepting birth control in their programs after this conference and committed to incorporating infertility treatment into programs for maternal and child health. Women in India have demonstrated a keen awareness of the links between fertility and infertility, even when they have not been joined in reproductive health services offered by the government. For example, an elderly woman informant in Tulsi Patel's study of fertility in a village in Rajasthan, Western India, offered both a critique of government reproductive health programs and power, saying, "If the government claims to be powerful enough to stop more children through those white-attired doctors, then why can't it provide children to those who are sterile and barren? It is only when it does so, can I believe in its superiority and power" (Patel 1994, 212). Although infertility services have begun to be offered in the public sector, most treatment still happens in private infertility clinics that charge much higher rates. Women being treated in the government hospitals in my study had usually consulted a gynecologist in private practice before visiting the government hospital and had often previously gone for treatment in other private clinics. For some, treatment in the government facility was the last resort after spending a great deal of money in private clinics without success.

Despite my initial hesitation about doing research in public facilities, following advice from Dr. Godrej and others, I moved on from small general clinics and private infertility clinics. Like many of the infertility patients I met later, after initial forays into the infertility "sector," I eventually found my way to two government hospitals offering specialized units or sections for infertility treatment. Even in these facilities, women seeking infertility treatment mingled to some extent with those who visited the hospital for other services, such as prenatal care, childbirth, birth control, abortion, and the care of premature infants. However, many women told me these were the first places they visited where they realized that they were not the only ones who could not conceive or could not sustain a pregnancy long enough to give birth to a live child. And while some of the clinical staff members—nurses and assistants—told me and them that there was no benefit (*fayda*) to be gained from hiding (*chupna* or *chupaana*) from the doctors, I saw women on numerous occasions try to hide their bodies from the medical gaze. I also heard staff criticize women for mixing other modes of healing and other local practices with biomedicine.

From physicians such as Dr. Ahmed and Dr. Godrej, I learned that physicians did know something about their patients' lives and problems. However, I also learned that their social positioning, medical consciousness, and interfaces with international organizations, as constituted through their particular experiences in India, powerfully influenced the ways they understood and ranked the range of options and compulsions (*majburi*, indicates lack of choice in difficult situations) facing people who sought their help for infertility problems. These initial interactions with physicians, before I spoke in detail with women visiting their clinics, helped me understand women's journeys. They also gave me reason to think about whether women might want to hide some aspects of their histories or reproductive quests from medical staff, and why.

One major appeal of biomedical clinical treatment with ARTs in India is that they offer people suffering from infertility the chance to fulfill their reproductive desires by creating children from their own gametes or to create the appearance of having done so. The Indian Council of Medical Research (ICMR) published ethical guidelines for ARTs and biomedical clinics that provide them (2005) as I was preparing for fieldwork, and debates in the Indian Parliament have gone on for many years. As is true in most countries, internal economic inequalities play a significant role in the stratification of access to reproductive technologies. Biomedical clinics in the private sector in India have dealt with some of these issues by instituting local programs for egg donation, whereby the recipient agrees to cover treatment expenses for the donor, who suffers from some other reproductive difficulty.

Other cultural studies of infertility in India (Bharadwaj 2016; Mulgaonkar 2001; Widge 2001) have been carried out in infertility clinics and have followed an approach similar to mine in this chapter: interviewing patients and medical staff and observing the general operations of the clinic. There are, however, some important differences. First, during the interim between their research in the late 1990s and mine, infertility clinics have proliferated throughout India. Whereas their studies were focused in two very large cities—New Delhi and Mumbai (Bombay)—and one smaller city—Jaipur (Rajasthan), mine was conducted entirely in Lucknow, which is significant as a center of Indo-Muslim culture and regional rural-to-urban migration.

In interviews with women undergoing fertility treatment in Lucknow, I found that their history of treatment tended to involve complex webs of movement—from countryside to city, from one area of the city to another, and from one type of practitioner to another—that generated an equally tangled web of paperwork that they more or less dutifully carried to the clinic. Some patients came with organized files of prior test results, medications, and procedures, often from other clinics, while others presented a pile of slips that they admitted was likely incomplete. Few women could make sense of the contents of the files on their own, and the medical staff generally gave them the minimally required information for obtaining and taking medicine or getting other procedures done. Since these instructions and prescriptions were usually written in English and in a hurried physician's hand, both language and technical terminology corroborated to make the files, slips, and receipts a collection of mostly secret knowledge to be collected and displayed to medical staff for interpretation and further direction about the course of treatment to be followed.

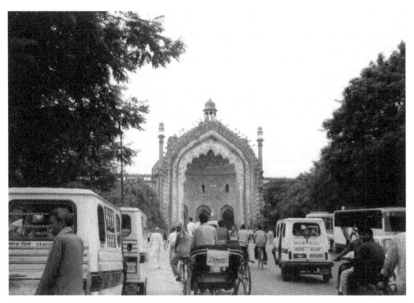

Figure 3.2. People speed by and through historic Lucknow spaces at all hours of the day and night. The Rumi Darvaza is situated near the Bara Imambara and many of the city's major medical facilities. (Photo by author.)

Both of the hospitals I worked in provide maternity care and general gynecological services, along with specialized infertility treatment. Among women I interviewed in these hospitals, sentiments such as "Be it a boy or a girl, one is necessary"; "At least there should be one [child]"; and, if pregnancy did not follow treatment, "There will be no family line [*vansh*], there will be no child [*aulad*]" were repeated to me many, many times.[4] Women came to the hospital with a variety of medical profiles and previous trajectories of treatment. They came from different areas of the city of Lucknow and from smaller cities, towns, and rural areas in central and eastern Uttar Pradesh. By appearance, they were Hindu and Muslim and belonged to more and less prosperous families. In Uttar Pradesh, diversity of dress and local accent is common, and this was true of the women who visited these two infertility clinics during the months I spent there. Nevertheless, as these women described dealing with fertility problems, many themes emerged that united their experiences across divisions of class, caste, and religion. Still, their abilities to pursue particular options for building their families ran against different limitations related to financial and familial factors.

Women who came to these hospitals trying to achieve pregnancy sometimes came alone; some were accompanied by their husbands or, occasionally, by other family members. In most cases, the hospital staff allowed me to sit with patients in a space more private than the general waiting room, where we could speak with relatively little interruption out of earshot of accompanying family members. Medical staff members marked their distance from women being seen in the clinic by their generally gruff manner in interactions with them. Some staff demonstrated annoyance toward women they saw in the clinic, especially when they struggled to answer questions about their medical history or their treatment reports. Once inside the rooms of the infertility unit, most women seemed relaxed and even eager to talk to pass the time between their exams and reports, in between episodes of scrutiny by the medical staff. Women's husbands sometimes accompanied them to respond to the medical staff's questions, then retreated to the waiting room, leaving their wives in comparative privacy. Women were generally curious and eager, or at least willing, to speak with me about their experiences. The vast majority of our interactions were conducted in the colloquial blend of Hindi and Urdu commonly spoken in central and eastern Uttar Pradesh. The speech of a few women reflected their rural residence in pronunciation and grammatical structure, but our conversations did not appear to suffer from my use of more standard Hindi/Urdu. A few women also launched into our conversations in English, and I followed their lead.

Women usually insisted that I talk with them together while they were waiting to be examined or to receive test results conducted that day, so our conversations sometimes had to be left

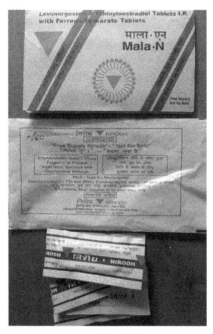

Figure 3.3. Examples of free contraceptives supplied at government
facilities, obtained from a public maternity hospital in Lucknow that also
offered infertility services. *Above,*
daily contraceptive pills. *Middle* and
lower, condoms. The common red
triangle identifies both as products
supplied through government programs. (Photo by author.)

unfinished. Most women were hurried and harried by the strains
of treatment, running among different hospital counters to register and submit fees or to purchase medicine and medical supplies,
such as syringes, ordered by the hospital doctors from the hospital shop or nearby medical stores. In addition to these details of
hospital treatment, some women were anxious to finish quickly
so their husbands could return to work, or so they could return
home to take care of their household chores of cooking, cleaning,

and caring for other family members. They were rarely allowed to be at ease in the clinical setting, where a nurse or "sister," a lower-level member of the clinical staff, might call for them or start giving them orders at a moment's notice.

In both hospitals, women entering the clinical space for examination had to either change their clothes or modify their dress. In the smaller hospital, women seeking infertility treatment were randomly interspersed with pregnant women having regular checkups throughout their pregnancies. I realized very quickly that the smaller hospital served a large number of Muslims when the *ayah* (āyah), a female assistant in the ultrasound room, shouted at patients repeatedly, "Take off your burqa! No burqas in the exam room!"[5] The full-length black veil worn by many Muslim women—and not by women of any other religious background—in Lucknow, especially in the old city, had to be removed before entering the small waiting area near the tiny room in which ultrasounds were conducted in the mornings. The *ayah*, a Hindu woman, would not tolerate women entering the exam space while veiled, even though it meant that those women would have to remove their burqas in the waiting room.

In this hospital and this part of the city, many, but certainly not all, Muslim women wore burqas, most often midcalf-length black gowns with a separate black headscarf worn in several styles, some covering their hair and entire face, except for their eyes, some simply framing the face like a bonnet. Others had a separate mesh or sheer black panel that covered even their eyes, which they would fling back over their foreheads when they needed to interact with someone or when they wanted a closer look at something. The waiting room was a bustling public place, where men, women, and children, young and old, sat waiting for their turn, their reports, or their family members who were being examined, drinking tea and eating while they waited. The *ayah* said that removing the burqa was a matter of hygiene because women wear their burqas everywhere—many, admittedly, looked a bit dusty—and because it would interfere with the ultrasound technician's ability to carry out the exam. Burqa-clad Muslim women were a common sight in this clinic, but they were certainly not the exclusive clientele. Unveiled Muslim women, as well as Hindus, Christians, and Sikhs, also visited the hospital for various procedures. In India, the burqa has often been seen by non-Muslims as a symbol marking the "otherness," "backwardness," and nonmodernity of Muslims, without appreciation for the nuances of meaning attributed to different styles of veils and veiling.

Women moved from the general waiting area into the small reception room and then onto the bed in the tiny ultrasound room where the ultrasound technician was often accompanied by two or more medical residents who recorded the ultrasound measurements and simultaneously received instruction in how to interpret the images on the grainy monitor. Women, many pregnant but some having their reproductive organs examined, laid on the exam table with their bellies bared while the technician asked them a few questions and conducted the ultrasound, in the process smearing their bellies with the clear jelly used to lubricate the transducer probe. The technician examined the green computer screen closely, measuring and making notes, then printed the results and passed them to the interns, who made any final notations before returning them to the women. Women were given basic information at this stage and sent to show the reports to their doctors. Time in the exam room was brief, while waiting for the examination and the results, securing the necessary receipts for payment, and showing the results to staff physicians easily occupied hours of patients' time.

Razia and Amina

On my first day at this clinic, the physicians on duty introduced me to two Muslim women who had come to the hospital for infertility treatment. After both assured me that they had no trouble understanding my speech and that there would be no need for a translator, the physicians departed to attend to their other duties, leaving us to talk. Razia, the wife of a rickshaw driver who stayed at home, told me about her infrequent menstrual cycles (*taarikh*) and about the taunts she sometimes heard in her in-laws' home about the absence of a child. Even though Razia said she was about twenty years old, she had already run away from an arranged marriage and had been in a love marriage for five years without giving birth. She pressured her husband to take her for investigation of infertility, but their small and inconsistent income meant significant disruptions in treatment. These gaps led to an otherwise needless repetition of tests and prevented any significant advances in dealing with whatever the problem might be.

The other woman, Amina, was in her early thirties. Although both of them were Muslims, the social differences between Razia and Amina were obviously vast. Amina told me that both she and her husband were involved in running businesses and had not even thought about children for the first few years of their marriage. When they realized that there might be some kind of fertility problem, they started treatment, and had been continuing it for about a year and a half, dealing with cysts and blockages in her fallopian tubes. Her journeys had taken her to Agra and Fatehpur Sikri to visit two Mughal-period sites in western Uttar Pradesh where people seek divine intercession in their fertility (and other) problems, and to a homeopathic doctor near her home in Lucknow.

On the day we met, she was due for a procedure to examine her fallopian tubes, which the attending *ayah* insisted I observe. Although Amina acted every bit a well-off, confident businesswoman, when the *ayah* asked her to remove her *shalwar*, the baggy pants underneath her tunic, Amina balked. Several male medical residents had entered the exam room to observe the procedure. Amina became shy and looked around anxiously. To me, her discomfort and fear seemed to fill the room, but the staff took no notice. The *ayah* scolded Amina for hesitating and asked, "How will the residents ever learn to perform such procedures if they aren't allowed to watch them?" Helplessly, Amina loosened her *shalwar* and laid down on the examination table. The physician entered the room and asked Amina to bend her knees and let her legs fall apart.

In my own extreme discomfort, to my chagrin, the *ayah* repeatedly called me closer to the exam table to better see what was happening, so that I, too, could learn. I only wanted to reassure Amina in her distress but felt unable to do so among the medical staff, who seemed to expect me to gaze with equal dispassion on the case before us. While Amina might have been able to hide the intimate details of her infertility treatment from those near and dear to her, she could not conceal herself from the strangers in the clinic. Inside the walls of the exam room, her vulnerability was on full display. After the procedure, she gathered herself together and left the area. I have not seen Amina since then, so I do not know whether she continued treatment at this hospital or elsewhere, nor whether or not she was able to conceive. She did say that she and her husband were open to adopting a child and mentioned an orphanage run by someone they knew in another part of the city. Amina's clinic encounter makes clear how extreme the contrasts of trying to obtain children through biomedical infertility treatment can be. In the world outside, women and their partners may go to extreme lengths to hide their bodies, their movements, and the particulars of their treatment from their families, friends, and neighbors, except as they find it necessary to reveal certain details in order to secure financial and material support. Inside clinics, the same women may find their bodies and their secrets more open and vulnerable than ever before in their lives.

At the larger, more specialized hospital, I noticed that women in burqas, and Muslim women in general, appeared much less frequently, even though both facilities were in parts of the city where many Muslims lived. Both Bharadwaj and Widge (2016, 2003; 2001) noted that in their late-1990s studies of fertility enhancement in biomedical fertility clinics in North India that advanced biomedical ARTs were used only by Hindus in the clinics where they conducted research. These studies suggested that Muslims may use other strategies for resolving their infertility, or that they abandon biomedical treatment sooner in the treatment process than Hindus. I would argue that the passage of time between studies plays a role in the level of acceptance of biomedical infertility treatment by Indian Muslims, but that other factors relating to minority status and particular understandings of Islamic law and Muslim custom also contribute to these differences. Several social activists I interviewed in Lucknow argued that Muslims avoid particular government hospitals because of the ill treatment they receive, which includes being categorized as "bad patients" and criticized about matters relating to fertility in particular. Some Muslims were using treatments available in biomedical clinics, but men, in particular, could also use other strategies to deal with their perceived lack of children, such as divorce and remarriage or adding another wife to an existing family.

In this facility, the infertility unit made up one part of an old, cavernous building dedicated to gynecological services. The unit in transition was just barely separate from the maternity section. The sections blended together in different ways from day to day, depending on how many women from the infertility unit needed cots to rest on after undergoing procedures and before leaving the hospital. This unit had its own ultrasound machine and staff members, including several *ayahs* (assistants), nurses, and laboratory staff who assisted with procedures. Machines and essential lights in the unit sometimes ran on backup power, while fans and other "nonessential" features ran only when the main electricity supply was operational. Running water also came and went, so staff members were prepared with alternative sources of water for basic needs.

The medical staff, doctors, and "sisters" (nurses and lower-level assistants) often referred to my conversations with women as "counseling," although I was careful to inform them that I was an anthropologist doing a research project for my PhD. Still, many women responded to me, at least initially, as they would in the role of patient, in ways that resembled their interactions with the

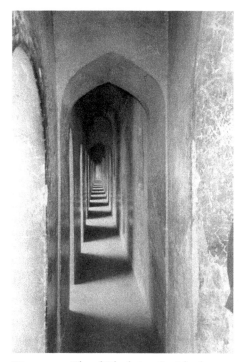

Figure 3.4. Bhool Bhulaiya: Inside the maze at Lucknow's eighteenth-century Bara Imambara. The site has religious uses, especially during Shi'a Muslim observances of Muharram, and is a magnet for tourists from Lucknow, across India, and around the world. The labyrinth inside is evocative of the many paths, distractions, and dead ends that may be part of fertility journeys. (Photo by author.)

medical staff. Some women gave me detailed reports of the "lady doctors" they had seen before coming to this clinic, and of their reproductive histories, which were usually an extended lament about money spent, medicine taken, and distances traveled, to no avail. A few had one living child but were unable to bear another—and would be identified by the medical staff as suffering from secondary infertility, perhaps resulting from an infection or a problem during the previous delivery. Some had conceived but suffered pregnancy loss—otherwise known as spontaneous abortion or miscarriage—one or more times. Others had never had a confirmed pregnancy, sometimes over years of marriage. A minority of women had used birth control early in their marriages and had only begun trying to conceive from six months to three years after their marriage. A few admitted to having undergone induced abortions (referred to as *safai* [cleaning] or *baccha giraana* [to cause the child to fall]) when they conceived very soon after marriage. Most had taken no concrete measures to prevent conception at any point after marriage. These women, whom I met multiple times during my research and their treatment, came from a variety of economic, caste, and religious backgrounds, and had diverse reproductive profiles. They shared, to a significant enough extent to subject themselves to the strain and expense of treatment, the hope that biomedical treatment would assist them in obtaining the children they desired.

The clinic's day-to-day activities included not only consultations between medical staff and patients, ultrasounds, and writing prescriptions but also procedures such as intrauterine insemination (IUI). In IUI, sperm collected either from the woman's partner or from a donor is injected into the patient's uterus by syringe. Physicians and other medical staff in the clinic referred to IUI as *pati ka paani pilaana* (to cause to drink/to irrigate with the husband's water), and several women stayed behind to wait for what sometimes felt like not only a practical arrangement because of the time involved but also like a ritual to conclude the clinical day. Women undergoing the procedure were called in together at the end of the day's course of treatment, usually by 1:00 pm, and laid close to one another while the medical staff carried out the procedure. Some of the staff chatted with women about their cases and histories in between giving them orders, using familiar terms of address—"breathe, close your legs, come down, open up (*kholo*)." The laboratory staff brought in needleless syringes containing the labeled semen samples and ceremoniously inserted them one by one, announcing the patient's name and creating a show of making sure that the right syringe got inserted into the right woman. The staff then placed pillows under the women's thighs while they lay with their legs straight out and crossed at the ankles for at least ten minutes before they were dismissed with instructions about when to return to the unit.

While women spent their time in the unit, many of their partners were tested elsewhere on the hospital premises. Medical staff rarely allowed husbands inside the unit, and those who were not being tested waited outside while their wives had tests or procedures done. During the time I spent there, the infertility unit was being remodeled and upgraded, and the unit moved from one temporary location to another. Women waited together in one room, where they changed clothes and took turns wearing one of the several green hospital gowns provided. One by one, they were called into the examination room to be seen by the medical staff and returned to await their results and further instructions. Most of my interactions with women took place in this room, neither a general waiting room nor an exam room. Women usually insisted that I speak with them together or one by one in the group, rather than isolate them for an interview, although much depended on the ebb and flow of patients. I agreed to this request. Others in the room listened more or less intently, and, on a few occasions, interactions became spirited group discussions.

MANAGING HOPE: EXPANDING AND CONTRACTING HORIZONS

From women I interviewed in infertility clinics, I heard stories of both harassment and support from in-laws. What I did not hear, in most cases, were completely overwrought, unrelenting narratives of despair. Mixtures of hope (*ummid* or *asha*) and realism emerged in women's narratives of their paths to this clinic and their evaluations of future possibilities. Despite the difficulties of undergoing treatment in a biomedical facility, trading surveillance by their in-laws for even more intimate surveillance by physicians and the compulsion to discipline their patterns of interaction with their husbands (intercourse was usually termed as *milna* or *milna-julna* [to meet] and was prescribed according to a schedule established by the doctor), for many women, treatment seemed to be a victory and proof of their worth in the marital household, a place where women's health often comes last.

Rama

Rama, a woman who had been trying to have a child for four years, had been coming to the clinic for three months after previously abandoning treatment. In her evaluation, "If it's in [my] destiny, then we'll get it [a child] . . . everybody wants children. Everyone's fond of them." While leaving responsibility for the outcome of treatment to fate, she did not reference the whims of destiny as a reason to abandon all action. She also said that coming to the clinic increased their hopes of success in getting a child and their desire to be successful. Like many women I met in the clinic, Rama had in-laws who supported her frequent trips to the clinic by taking care of the household chores in her absence. The sentiment that coming to the clinic increased one's hopes but also increased desire, sometimes to the point of desperation, was also often expressed by women in the English fertility clinics studied by Sarah Franklin in the late 1980s and early 1990s (1997, 183). Franklin describes in vitro fertilization (IVF) as a "hope technology" (1997, 202–203) that demands much balance, saying, "IVF presents contradictory demands: to hope enough but not too much; to try your best but realize it is a gamble; to make sense of the unexplained; to believe in miracles" (1997, 191). Hindi/Urdu offers a plethora of ways to express uncertainty and the limited control of actors on the outcome of their efforts, from the subjunctive mood that grammatically indicates possible futures, to constructions such as *inshallah* or *bhagvan kare* (god-willing) that often bracket statements about the future in everyday speech. These constructions do not indicate complete fatalism, nor do they provide complete comfort about the ability to bring about a particular outcome.

Shivani

Oscillations between sadness and hope, frustration and desires for the future were evident in women's stories of their treatment. I met Shivani in the ninth month of treatment when she was about to undergo IUI for the sixth time at the government clinic, after she had abandoned treatment at a private hospital because of the excessive expense. She had not been pregnant in nearly three years of marriage and said that along with going to the clinic, she took comfort from her mother-in-law, had consulted a *pandit* (Brahmin religious specialist), and was fasting every Monday in honor of the god Shiva. Her words were both mournful and hopeful. She started out saying, "I've become distressed . . . it hurts. . . . It's a very bad experience. Let it not be so with any- one [use of subjunctive/conditional verb]." As our conversation continued, she said that many people asked about her children, without thinking whether or not they should ask. She said that she thought about adopting a child, preferably an unknown out- sider, with no attachment to any other extended family members. Her husband, she said, would prefer to have their "own" child, and encouraged her by saying that they hadn't been going for treatment for very long; it was still possible that they would get a child this way. If it's not possible, she said, then they would adopt, but not just yet—"When I/we get exhausted. Right now I/we still have courage (*himmat*)."

Mamta

During my time in the clinic, the most emotionally distressed and, for me, most distressing woman I encountered was not a young daughter-in-law unable to conceive but a Brahmin (high- caste Hindu) woman in her midthirties who had begun coming to the clinic for treatment one year earlier, following the death of her only son after a paralysis attack at the age of seventeen. Her appearance, her manner of speaking, and the formality with which she addressed me, along with her words, communicated her status as a struggling lower-middle-class woman from a rural background with relatively little education to help her navigate the ins and outs of clinical infertility treatment. Even now, recalling her countenance and her narration gives me chills.

Mamta's story tumbled out of her unbidden before I could compose myself or the head nurse could ask me to leave this poor woman alone. She told me (*memsahib* [ma'am]) to take notes as I needed to, describing the loss of her son, how she had never used any birth control, yet he was the only one. She said the physicians had diagnosed a hormonal problem. Becoming visibly emotional, she said that God gave him and took him back and that if she could have done anything, she would have sold her land, her house, her jewelry, everything. Following the death of her son, she stayed home and refused to wear jewelry or celebrate festivals. "We are without support [emotional and/or financial, *besahara*, besahārā] . . . when you don't have someone of your own, no one else comes to take their place." By coming to the clinic, she was hoping "that my *bhaiyya* [affectionate term for her son] might come back [subjunctive verb]." Only if the treatment did not work would they consider any alternative. Her use of the word *besahara* to describe the family's condition goes far beyond the provision of economic resources. It signifies an even more profound precarity of existence—the specter of loneliness, and of the absence of kin on which elderly parents might rely not only for care but also for companionship and assurance of a future for the family that could serve as emotional consolation in old age. Mamta was deeply disturbed by her experiences, and the clinic seemed to be the only place that could offer hope of remedying her terrible loss. Whether her display had become disruptive to the unit, or because she had become so visibly upset by telling the story, I cannot say for certain, but the head nurse soon asked me not to follow up in detail with Mamta.

The government clinics where I conducted fieldwork did not distribute any printed information to people undergoing infertility treatment. They did not advertise the clinic or their rates of success. Conversations with the staff and with women seeking treatment made it clear that women commonly began treatment only to abandon it due to emotional exhaustion, frustration, or financial difficulty. The head nurse at the large clinic also stated that women who became pregnant after being treated at the clinic frequently disappeared, so the staff never found out the treatment's ultimate result. These women, she argued, wanted to conceal having undergone infertility treatment, and so would cut off contact with the unit once a pregnancy was established. As government institutions, the clinics did not have a clear financial incentive to follow up with former patients or to generate strong statistical data to present to prospective patients. As with the Papua New Guinea hospitals in Alice Street's (2012, 45) account, struggles between hope for transformation and resignation to failure also played out in these Indian hospitals. However, the hope mostly lay with women seeking infertility treatment, and the resignation to failure, with the hospital staff. Staff members knew about the low odds for successful treatment, but they also knew from experience that many women would disappear during treatment. Whether their absence signaled lack of funds, despair over lack of success, or, indeed, a successful pregnancy and birth, staff resigned themselves to knowing little about their patients' long-term outcomes once they disappeared from the clinic.

On the other hand, private clinics I visited had strong reasons to promote the success of their practice by encouraging prospective patients with pamphlets that featured opening lines such as "Keeping hopes alive" and "Test tube babies: many have come, many more to come." For example, Dr. Kapoor, who led the patient education session described in chapter 2, told me that her

clinic held a party every year for the families of the test-tube babies born with her help. Throughout my research, many people
mentioned this high-profile physician when I told them of my
interests. She had clearly built a strong private practice and also
had significant exposure in the local media. Her clinic's materials
highlighted the low success rate in cases of IVF and intracytoplasmic sperm injection, and she frankly evaluated the options
of people suffering from infertility. In her patient-education class,
she listed all the procedures performed and the costs for each
and did not mince words about the difficulties of pursuing treatment or the limitations of health and financial resources. Yet Dr.
Kapoor also did not advocate that people suffering from infertility give up hope and accept their childless state, concluding her
sessions by arguing that "baby *zarur hona chahie*" (you should
definitely have a baby), even if the baby were adopted. After all
the talk I had heard about concealing infertility treatment from
families and other prying eyes, I was surprised to see newspaper
clippings and promotional pamphlets in which Dr. Kapoor posed
for photographs with families created through IVF, both parents
and children.

NORTH INDIAN "HOPE TECHNOLOGIES"
FOR CHILDREN AND FAMILIES

Women in infertility clinics often recited to me the places they
had visited in the hopes of conceiving a child, including gynecologists' offices, biomedical clinics, and nonbiomedical healing
sites. From both Hindus and Muslims, I learned of local sites,
including Hindu and Muslim shrines, where women could make
offerings. For example, at the grave of a Muslim holy person (a
mazaar), women offer cotton or silk bedsheets embroidered with
metallic thread (*chaadar*), flowers, cardamom pods, and sweets
(especially *revri*). At some sites, women would tie a thread (*dagha
bandhna*) to a tree or other sacred object and make their wish or

vow, promising to return to untie the thread and make a special offering if their wish were fulfilled. Famous sites such as Ajmer Sharif, the shrine, or *dargah*, of medieval Sufi master Hazrat Moinuddin Hasan Chishti in Rajasthan, Western India, and sites at Agra/Fatehpur Sikri, Uttar Pradesh, associated with Mughal ruler Akbar, also appeared in women's lists of places one might go in search of the blessings needed to obtain a child.

Other women mentioned Hindu holy men (*tantriks, babas,* or *pandits*) from whom they might take advice or medicine, or whose advice had been sought by other family members on their behalf. One Hindu woman said that her mother-in-law had brought her medicine from a *tantrik*, but she refused to take it and she had never visited that sort of holy person herself because she did not believe in them. Another Hindu woman said that her mother-in-law got a *taaviz*, a protective amulet filled with a small piece of paper inscribed with Qur'anic verses, made for her. She said that she wore the *taaviz*, although she herself did not believe in its power. This woman did not, however, express any discomfort about being given an amulet containing Quranic verses. She framed her rejection of its efficacy not as a rejection of Islam but as an affirmation of her belief in the power of biomedicine, and as an affirmation that while wearing such a ritual object could not harm her prospects for becoming pregnant, it would please her mother-in-law.

Muslim women I interviewed often said that they would not consult an expert in religious law about their appropriate course of treatment because they considered this to be a doctor's area of expertise. However, many clearly expressed the social concern that babies should be conceived only with the husband's sperm because the paternity of the resulting child should not be questioned. Although polygyny is theoretically a legal option for Muslim men—but not for Muslim women or people from other religious backgrounds—it was not a strategy used among people I met. Threats of marital dissolution (*talaq*, talāq) or bringing another wife into the household served mostly as ways for a man's parents, and especially his mother, to cajole their sons' wives into producing children. Both inside and outside of clinics, women from different religious backgrounds consistently argued that the experience of infertility overrides religious allegiances. I heard again and again that women facing the prospect of childlessness had common experiences of exploitation and family strife, and that while they might do so quietly, women disregarded religious boundaries in their quests for children, even as they might respect and uphold them in other areas of daily life. However, economic and religious factors limited the medical and other options that women could hope to pursue in their search for children.

Women volunteered information about multiple strategies for overcoming infertility when I asked them what people might do in cases of infertility other than going to an infertility clinic, and/or what they had done, if anything, but this was not the first information they volunteered about their fertility journeys. In clinics, these nonbiomedical strategies generally only entered conversation after women completed their narrations of the different gynecologists and infertility clinics they visited in their villages, nearby towns, and/or cities in Uttar Pradesh. Physicians and other medical staff generally discounted and even ridiculed such multiple strategies by women as a waste of money, as superstition, and as markers of their failure to embrace "modern" life. Physicians might recognize amulets or other jewelry worn by women as indications that they had visited holy people and comment on it. Few women I met in infertility clinics objected to these strategies; some disavowed their own faith in them while accepting them from family members. If these strategies did not succeed in bringing a child into their lives, at least they might bind family members closer together.

Medical staff asked women detailed questions about their medical history in order to complete a standardized form that became a permanent part of their record of treatment at the clinic.

This file would slowly fill with the results of tests and catalogs of procedures, ultrasound reports, prescribed medicines, and other treatment details. Interviews to ascertain medical history bore some similarities to questions I asked women; however, physicians generally did not ask whether patients had visited practitioners of Ayurveda or Unani medicine, or other healers or holy people. Depending on the physician, any of these practitioners might be included under Dr. Godrej's category of "quacks," although the term most commonly refers to village practitioners with significant experience and/or family history of serving in healing roles, but without formal medical credentials. Many physicians dispensed with such questions and considered these histories irrelevant to the course of treatment in biomedical clinics unless their examination showed some type of damage that might be traced to a previous intervention.

HOPING TO BECOME MOTHERS, WAITING FOR AULAD

The vast majority of the women I met who were suffering from infertility were still hoping to fulfill their desire to become mothers by giving birth to their own child and to avoid having to think about the decision to either accept their childless state or to take another course of action in order to bring children into their homes. In 2005–07, I placed less emphasis on the perspectives of older childless women, and I also encountered difficulties in getting introductions to such women. Even when friends or contacts knew of such individuals or couples, they were hesitant to introduce me and the topic to them, whether because of the awkwardness of raising what might be a sensitive topic or because it might bring into relief awareness of the individual's or couple's childless state in a way that would normally remain in the background. In reflections on narrative in her research on women and infertility in Kerala, South India, Catherine Kohler Riessman posits that the oldest women in her study, who were in their forties and rather unlikely to conceive, constructed themselves as complete persons without children, although they often positioned themselves within worlds that included children, even though they could not claim them as biologically their "own" (2002, 162, 165–66). In all three of the narratives Riessman analyzed, the women were still with their husbands, although in one case, the end of the marriage seemed to be a distinct possibility if children did not materialize. In this very small sample, Riessman offered an optimistic view of the ultimate reconciliation of married women to the state of childlessness, and their potential to present themselves as full women with full lives, even without a claim to motherhood.

Because I worked with women suffering from infertility who sought treatment in government clinics, I was able to talk with women from a broad range of socioeconomic backgrounds. However, I found out very little in terms of concrete reports of the outcome of women's quests to become mothers. In private clinics like Dr. Kapoor's, tracking the progress of particular couples' outcomes formed a significant part of the work required to promote the clinic's status and to recruit future patients. Unlike in Dr. Kapoor's clinic, government clinics had no brochures with smiling babies, no parties for families created using ARTs. The future of these clinics depends on government funding, not on publicity, and staff salaries are on a fixed scale not tied to treatment outcomes. Clinical staff said they usually did not know what happened to the women, whether they had been successful in becoming pregnant, or whether they had decided to either discontinue treatment or to pursue treatment at a different facility. Regarding the confidentiality of people pursuing infertility treatment and given the secrecy that most people maintained around their treatment regimen, perhaps this was a sensible course of inaction. It does go against the recommendations of the ICMR, which advocates that clinics try to determine treatment outcome by providing patients with a response form to return to the clinic and counseling them about the importance of the form (ICMR 2005, 62). The guidelines offered by the ICMR about the regulation of ART clinics have the potential to shape the practice of assisted reproductive medicine throughout India, but they are not legally enforceable, so it is up to clinics to decide whether or not to abide by these recommendations. The result is that many women's stories of attempting to solve their infertility through treatment at biomedical clinics remain hurried and half-told, even if someone asks or cares to listen, of which there is no guarantee. Clinics do not universally offer counseling, even though the ICMR also recommends that people seeking treatment be offered such counseling (ICMR 2005, 22–23, 58).

In Lucknow, most women who talked to me about the importance of becoming mothers and how women could become mothers in cases of reproductive difficulty were extremely hesitant to consider any method that involved the introduction of a new family member who did not share the same "blood" (*khun*) or background as the rest of the family. This could refer to some form of adoption, fostering, or the use of new reproductive technologies involving, for example, donated ova or sperm. Women expressed these hesitations both in reference to their own viewpoints and as an indication of what "society" (*samaj*) considered to be appropriate or inappropriate reproduction. They worried whether or not other extended family members would accept the child as their own, and whether the child would grow to see themself as a true part of the family. Issues of inheritance and loyalty to the family were relevant here, but more challenging to me was the idea that the child's "blood" could be a barrier to their adjustment in the household, a reason that could be cited for fostering or adopting a child from within one's extended family—the match would be right because of the similar family background of the child. My own field data speaks most clearly to the extended liminal state of women hoping to become mothers, the in-between-ness of trying to find a way to produce *aulad*. Waiting for *aulad* could delay the possibility of exercising other options for seeking children. These concerns gave women pause about considering unconventional methods of reproduction, including the use of donated gametes to create their future children. They did not universally dissuade women from pursuing such options, but they did drive women to secrecy about just what happened in the clinic.

TRYING: HOPING, WAITING, HIDING

Women who sought infertility treatment in government facilities during my research period in Lucknow came from a variety of backgrounds that influenced their treatment experiences. In the context of the clinic, women were deferential toward the medical staff yet quite free in speaking with me, in ways that might not have been possible had I interacted with them in their homes, with family members present, or with a translator. These women overwhelmingly asserted that biomedical treatment as carried out by infertility specialists was their best hope for conceiving children. However, many of them also visited a variety of holy places or people at different points in their search for children. Few women totally discounted these sites as possibly efficacious, although they often expressed skepticism about the power of these places and people and the substances obtained from them to bring about the birth of a child. I attribute this skepticism partly to the increasing influence of biomedicine and science in general in urban South Asia and to the biases of women using biomedical treatment in the hopes of overcoming infertility problems.

Women in clinics who got strong support from husbands or other family members exuded confidence, even though they were regularly subjected to procedures that violated their norms of modesty and bodily comfort. Despite long litanies of treatment failures, high expenditure of resources, and the prolonged inconvenience of travel for treatment, most women still expressed measured hope for the success of their efforts. Overwhelmingly, women expressed the hope that they would find success in the clinic and would not have to resort to adoption—as they put it, taking someone else's child to raise as their own—in order to attain their goal of becoming mothers. Still, most of them were realistic enough about their chances to know that, in the end, they might not get children through infertility clinics. Only then would most of these women, who because of their relative privilege and success in managing family relationships had been able to pursue their quests for children in biomedical infertility clinics, consider other options for creating families. In the process of pursuing biomedical infertility treatment, they gained unique opportunities to build their relationships with their husbands and to position themselves as highly valued family members because of their access to biomedical methods for resolving infertility, while hiding the details of their family-making excursions.

NOTES

1. All names of medical staff and women suffering from infertility in this chapter are pseudonyms.

2. I have listed round figures here to protect the clinic's confidentiality and identity.

3. Under the Pre-Natal Diagnostic Techniques (Regulation and Prevention of Misuse) Act 1994 and Amendment Act 2002 (Patel 2007a).

4. Quotations from interviews I conducted in Lucknow in infertility clinics and meetings in various spaces from 2005 to 2007. This chapter also includes excerpts from and references to my fieldnotes and journal entries composed during the same time.

5. The term *ayah* generally means a children's nurse or ladies' maid.

FOUR

REPRODUCTIVE REALITIES

Managing Inequality

You'll find plenty of kids in Gehumandi, in the market. To some
people, God has given no children, not even one. And to some
people He's given children, lots and lots of children.

—Group conversation participant, Gehumandi,
Lucknow, 2007

GHAR CHALAANA: TO KEEP THE HOME RUNNING

Gehumandi was a fairly large but ramshackle settlement (*basti*)
situated in the heart of the old city of Lucknow, within walking
distance of the city's most famous historical monuments.[1] According to residents, most of the people living there were Sunni
Muslims who had migrated from rural eastern Uttar Pradesh
to work in the city, some as long as fifteen to twenty years ago.
Although these residents were relative newcomers to Lucknow,
Muslims in general are not new to the city of Lucknow, to the
state of Uttar Pradesh, or to India.

A large proportion of Gehumandi residents were artisans who
worked in the textile industry, taking on various roles in producing garments, such as stitching the *chikan* and *zardozi* hand embroidery that makes textiles from Lucknow famous across India

and around the world.[2] During a visit to the *basti* with workers from a local nongovernmental organization (NGO), women
showed me elaborate pieces on which they had completed some
part of the work. One young woman told me that she was given 50
paise (1/2 rupee, or about 1 cent) for each small net design that she
made on a garment—her specialty, and one that could earn her
20 rupees (about 40 cents at the time) on an intricate *kurta*, the
long, loose top worn over trousers—but that she should get more.
In between completing their household duties and looking after
small children, women stitched on handheld looms to supplement the family's income. Muslim women in Uttar Pradesh often
take on home-based work that allows them to earn money while
looking after children, without attracting the criticism from family and others that working outside the home can bring. In some
homes in Gehumandi, looms stretched tight with brightly col-
ored saris filled the front room, while several boys and men surrounded the cloth, each completing a part of the extremely fine,
delicate embroidery work with gold- or silver-tinged thread. The
brilliant colors of the pristinely clean and pressed fabric embel-
lished with intricate hand-stitched designs struck me as a grand
contrast to the drab surroundings of the lanes of the *basti* and the
dark interiors of both homes and the NGO office. Although educational posters filled the walls, the office itself was constructed
from similar mud, bamboo, and hay as the homes surrounding it.

In Lucknow, I have been fortunate to be introduced to Muslim women who were involved in many different pursuits. The
ones other community members looked to as prominent leaders
and "worth meeting" were often women from well-established,
wealthy families who had few worries about their family's financial status and pursued a variety of social causes.[3] Such women
were quite highly educated and well-spoken and were certainly
much more bold, forthright, and confident than I was at the time.
I initially came into contact with most of these women one way
or another through my connections with Urdu language and lit-

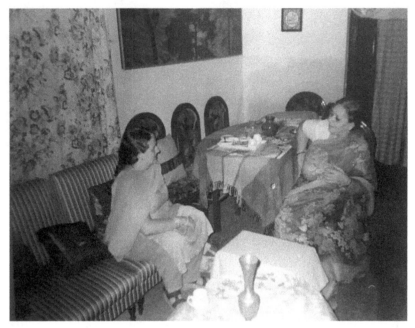

Figure 4.1. Chai and chat with teacher, Urdu scholar, and friend Dr. A. Y. Mohsin in Lucknow. (Photo by author.)

erature. Most people in India now associate Urdu with Muslims, with cultural elites of the past, and with poetry and films. In everyday speech, Urdu may sound just like Hindi, or it may drip with ornamental elements that lead people to characterize Urdu as a flowery, "sweet language" (*meethi zabaan*). In any case, my interests in Urdu connected me with networks of Muslim women in Lucknow. As I explained that my research related to women's health, I discovered that several of the women I met were involved in health-related activities or knew someone who was and invited me to see them at work. While some people I met in India thought studying Urdu to be a useless pursuit, it was Urdu that provided an entry point for me to observe the operations of several charitable organizations that provided free or lost-cost health services primarily to low-income Muslims in Lucknow.

This chapter focuses on how women living in one poor neighborhood in Lucknow struggled to negotiate the challenges of
creating and maintaining healthy families in difficult living conditions. By examining interactions in low-cost health camps organized by an Islamic charity and among women from the *basti*
(a theoretically temporary, often unauthorized settlement) community that primarily used the health camp's services, I show
how both access to resources and the prejudices of health workers shape women's abilities to fulfill their reproductive desires.
I highlight the tenuous nature of reproduction among Muslims
living in the *basti*, even among those who do not suffer from infertility. For people suffering from infertility and the social effects
of childlessness, the successful conception and birth of a child is
the main focus of their efforts. Still, it is only a beginning step to
successfully producing *aulad*, a tentative process that is magnified in significance for people living in poverty, whose conditions
of life give them no guarantee of survival, much less of privacy at
any stage in reproduction. In this context, even people who do
not encounter difficulties in conceiving and birthing children
have no assurance of successful reproduction as they define it.

The two health-related organizations I dealt with most closely
in Lucknow operated in different ways. One, which I call Millat,
focused exclusively on providing low-cost health visits and medicine to women and children. The other, which I call Andolan,
dedicated most of its resources to education and economic empowerment, but it also addressed health issues. The two organizations shared one important feature: they both worked primarily
with people living in a single *basti* community in the old city of
Lucknow, Gehumandi. The weekly health camp organized by
Millat was held in a spacious hall a couple of kilometers away
from the settlement. Although the camp did not restrict attendance to people living there, a large proportion of patients at the
camp cited Gehumandi as their place of residence. Andolan had
an office within the *basti* settlement, which served as the focal

point of the NGO's activities. Andolan also worked primarily with women and children on various ways to promote educational advancement and economic empowerment. The leaders of Andolan were well-connected with other networks of social activists, and they frequently organized seminars in collaboration with other NGOs, which some Gehumandi residents who participated in the NGO's activities also attended. In part, my networks in Lucknow drew me to these organizations and to a connection with a Muslim majority neighborhood and might be termed an ethnographic choice. However, recent work on religion and poverty in India also suggests that being identifiably Muslim increases the chances of living with poverty and discrimination.

A literature far too large to discuss here describes Muslims entering India well over a thousand years ago and the conversions, conflicts, cocreation, and coexistence that have followed. This literature also comes with deep and shifting politics over religion and citizenship, secularism and its critics in post–independence India, and a host of other topics. When taken as a unified category—and this act itself is a matter of significant debate, since it flattens the diversity of Muslims living in India—Muslims comprise approximately 14 percent of India's total population (Ghosh and Singh 2015).[4] Historically, more Muslims have tended to live in North India than in the south, and that still holds true, although migrations of Muslims to Pakistan, and Sikhs and Hindus to India at the partition that created independent India and Pakistan in 1947 and since then have shifted the concentration and distribution of people identified by religious categories. In Uttar Pradesh, as of the 2001 census, about 18.5 percent of residents were counted as Muslim.[5] In Lucknow, that proportion rises. However, the cultural influence of Muslims, of Islamic religion, and of Islamicate culture—practices and cultural products of Muslims that are not explicitly religious (Hodgson 1974)—far outstrips the number of residents identified as Muslim. A glance at internet resources on "religion and population in India" reveals the political tensions involved in the collection and analysis of these demographic characteristics of contemporary India, particularly regarding changes in population by religion (see Singh 2020).

Muslims living in Lucknow talk about a variety of factors that distinguish different groups. Among these are Sunni or Shi'a affiliation; belonging to different caste-like groups that influence marriage decisions, such as Sayyid, Pathan, or Qasai; landholding status and village links; educational status; being conversant with different local varieties of Hindi/Urdu, literary Urdu, and/or English; and gender. In terms of Lucknow's culture and heritage, Muslim influence extends far beyond any accounting of population in numbers. In present-day Lucknow, long-established, wealthy cultural elites and poor rural migrants may both be identified as Muslim. They may (or may not) embrace similar religious practices. They inhabit the world quite differently but may be brought together in any number of ways, as employer and employee; as patron and beneficiary, as in the health camps I describe in this chapter; as members of social organizations; or as fellow worshippers. The hierarchical nature of many of these encounters should be apparent, and it is crucial to the contexts of reproduction included in this chapter.

From the homes and lanes of Gehumandi and other nearby localities, women arrived at the Millat health camp by foot, in shared motorized tempos, or by bicycle rickshaw, toting along their children and sick female relatives and friends. The camp ran one morning a week, and some women seemed to turn up every week to keep themselves and their children going. Millat funded basic health services largely through donor funds given as *zakat* (zakāt), a required gift—generally 2.5 percent of excess wealth, depending on the nature of that wealth—for the poor, which most Muslims give around the time of Eid-ul-Fitr at the end of the fasting month of Ramadan (also known in North India as Ramzan). In addition, Millat was also locally known to provide financial assistance to people in extreme distress and to help with the fees required to send poor children to local schools. Volunteers at the health camp were charged with overseeing the distribution of these funds. They had their own ideas about how the money would best be spent. They often preached to the women who came with requests and exerted their own influence on the flow of resources. For the most part, Millat's volunteers portrayed themselves not as feminists fighting for women's equality but as people dedicated to helping the poor survive. To promote survival within the restrictions of limited resources, they often suggested practical strategies that reinforced gender discrimination, such as choosing to fund a son's education over a daughter's or scolding a poor woman to take up domestic work in more wealthy peoples' homes to support her family.

Around the time of the Eid-ul-Fitr celebration, special distributions of food and other donated items were also given to people who regularly turned up the health camp. So, in addition to getting help with minor ailments, as well as the potential for referrals and monetary help in getting more serious ailments treated at other medical facilities, attendees also stood to benefit in other ways from their long-term association with Millat. For regular visitors, Millat could be an important support for their household, and a significant help in keeping the house running: *ghar chalaana*. Running the household means providing financial support, but it also means keeping the people of the house, the *ghar waale*, well enough to continue with their work. People who showed up at the health camp at Eid time, or when the new school term was starting, but otherwise never visited the camp would likely be turned away empty-handed by Millat volunteers.

Volunteers sat at a desk in the large hall, in between the small room where doctors saw patients and the dispensary where one or both of two sisters who had benefited from educational opportunities provided by Millat dispensed the medicines. On an average morning, volunteers registered over one hundred patients. At Eid time, twice as many people might appear, completely overwhelming the capacity of the volunteers, most of whom were elderly women retired from professional positions. Women stood in a long line in the large hall waiting for their turn to pay 5 rupees, a little more than 10 cents, to get a *parcha* (parchā), a small slip of paper that entitled them to see a doctor. Most of the doctors and the young women who staffed the pharmacy, commonly referred to as the dispensary, each received a small payment of 80–100 rupees (about $1.75 to $2.25) from the fees collected from patients. For physicians, it was a trifling sum compared to what they received for seeing patients in private practice, which could range from 10 rupees to 500 or more per patient, depending on the locality; the doctor's specialty; and other factors, such as how elaborate their facilities were and how much crowd the doctor's reputation garnered. Still, the Millat doctors gathered the money they received, usually in small change, which they appreciated because it could come in handy for short rickshaw rides and small purchases. I have also hoarded small change in India, as it can be hard to come by and can be indispensable for buying milk for evening tea, getting a good deal on vegetables, and buying other small items from vendors who may not have the cash to change a large bill.

Doctors used the patients' *parchas* to write notes about each patient's examination and to prescribe medicine. Patients often reused these slips of paper from one week to the next, and volunteers noted the new date on the old slip when they received fees for that day's checkup. A single *parcha* frequently carried records of several checkups by multiple doctors. Moreover, patients kept and carried the slips—folded up inside their purses, their clothes, or tattered plastic bags—and stored them in their meager homes. By the time a *parcha* became filled with the records of previous ailments, it bore the wounds of carriage and storage, yellowed, wrinkled, and much worse for the wear. Still, volunteers hesitated to provide a fresh slip of paper for each visit.

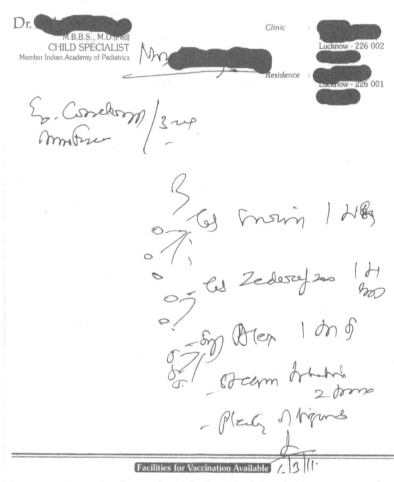

Figure 4.2. Example of a *parcha* with physician's handwritten notes and prescription. (Photo by author.)

Dr. Rehana / Rehana baji

When I first began to attend the health camp, one of the places where I observed the operations was from behind a desk. This was where Millat member Rehana baji, the quietly dignified, regal, elderly Muslim woman and doctor of social science who first introduced me to the organization, kept busy filling in

parchas, taking money, and making change.[6] She also asked after the women's families and made other general inquiries that
demonstrated her long involvement with the women and the
organization. Rehana baji always wore a sari and glasses and
scrupulously covered her head with the end of her sari when
she felt it appropriate, such as when she heard the call to prayer
(*azan*, azān) or when she interacted with male Muslim scholars.
She was graceful and full of humility, yet fierce in setting forth
her views. Extremely well-read in English and Urdu literature and
Islamic scholarship, she seemed at ease with people at every level
of society. She sometimes, however, became visibly emotionally
distressed by the persistent pleas of people attending the health
camp, which continued even as she walked the few steps to the
small car in which her driver waited to shuttle her and other volunteers home. Despite her high level of formal education, Rehana
baji expressed discomfort with reading Hindi script (Devana-
gari), and she sometimes asked me to read letters or forms women
brought with them as part of their requests for help, especially
with school fees for their children.

As I became a regular visitor at the camp, I also took on duties
of *parcha* maker, asking women the standard questions: name,
age, place of residence. Some women either did not know their
ages, actively concealed them, or subtracted years by saying, "I
don't know" or "Just write 40." Rehana baji liked to chide them,
saying, "Your son can't be less than 30 years old, and you call
yourself 40?" A majority of the women listed Gehumandi as their
place of residence, although some would give answers like "along
the river side" or "under the bridge." While some women would
get new *parchas*, others would pull out old, wrinkled, folded-up
parchas in some stage of decay from their *shalwar kameez* (tunic
and pants) or from somewhere inside the folds of a burqa. They
would pay 5 rupees to have a new date entered on the *parcha* so
they could see the doctor again, whether to continue previous
treatment or to discuss a new ailment. Although some women

thought that having the *parcha* from their previous appointment, no matter how ancient, entitled them to a free return visit, volunteers insisted that they needed the current date entered on the *parcha*, and for that, they must submit the required fees. Once in a while, though, the volunteers took pity on someone and let her go without paying.

Volunteers, doctors, and patients were nearly all Muslim women and their children, except for one male doctor, who was trained in Unani medicine.[7] According to the volunteers, patients favored him because of how he interacted with them and perhaps because of his tendency to prescribe medicine more freely than the other physicians. Volunteers sometimes drew attention to religion in their interactions with patients, mostly by asking them questions such as "Have you taught your child to say his (or her) prayers?" and then nodding with approval as the children dutifully recited them. Doctors also referenced religion at times, especially in matters relating to childbirth. Although the health camp made no specific restrictions on eligibility by religion, it was a religiously based organization funded primarily by charitable donations of Muslims. Hindus did occasionally come for examination, and they were given the same treatment as other patients. However, the decidedly Islamic orientation and membership of the organization and the location of the camp in a building belonging to another Islamic group attracted mostly Muslims. The composition of the surrounding neighborhoods in terms of religious background and preconceptions on the part of prospective patients about who would be accepted for treatment may also have contributed to the demographics of visitors to this particular camp.

Once women acquired the precious *parcha* with an entry for the current date, they would wait to meet with either the group of women doctors who sat together in a small room to the side of the main hall and examined patients together or one by one simultaneously, with multiple conversations going on at the same time, or to the male doctor, who sat in one corner of the main hall. The male doctor was quite jovial and entertained seated patients while conducting examinations and prescribing medicine. In the room where the other doctors sat, women generally stood up with their children, if they had them along, while the doctors sat around the desk. Examinations consisted of a statement by the patient about the problem that brought them in, whether it was their own or their child's, followed by a period of questions and answers between doctor and patient. Occasionally, the doctor listened for the patient's pulse or asked them to check their weight on the small bathroom scale kept in one corner of the room.

Physical contact between doctor and patient was minimal, and patients stuck out their tongues and displayed injuries on command, while the doctors examined them by sight at some distance. The social, educational, and economic distance between doctor and patient always felt palpable to me. Doctors freely commented on the cleanliness of the women and their children and the conditions in which they lived, quite frankly disparaging them with questions such as "Don't you ever bathe him? Of course he'll get sick. How will his body not erupt with boils?" and then giving them instructions about how to bathe the children. Sometimes they went as far as giving out bars of soap or 5 or 10 rupees, scolding the mothers to bathe their children regularly and thoroughly. Such boils (*daane*) were common ailments among the children, along with complaints of fever (*bukhar*), cold (*zukaam*), general listlessness (*susti*), and diarrhea (*dast*), and the pharmacy was stocked with various tonics and pills, both allopathic (biomedical pharmaceuticals) and Ayurvedic, to remedy these problems. One of the doctors, Dr. Razia, was particularly zealous in distributing medicine and ordered patients to get the medicine from the counter and then show it to her. She explained the method of dosing and then wrote on the outer box or the bottle. She told me this would prevent women from returning or reselling the medicine to another pharmacy, instead of taking it themselves or giving it to their child.

In general, the female doctors' manner resembled that of disdainful caretakers who repeatedly dispensed advice knowing that, at best, their patients would half-follow it. While their affect magnified the social distance between doctor and patient and denoted poor patients as "other," doctors used other methods of emphasizing their connections with patients. They frequently referenced their common religion and the tenets of it that could be cited as an inspiration for health practices that aligned with the doctors' priorities. They mentioned cleanliness as a prerequisite to proper religious conduct and encouraged women to give up vices that were not only religiously dubious, such as chewing tobacco, but also—according to the doctors—a poor use of their scarce financial resources that could be better put to use supporting their children's education or buying nutritious foods.

Women complained of some of the same ailments that afflicted their children, but they also reported problems linked to their reproductive health. Regardless of the nature of their complaint, doctors asked when their last menstrual period took place and how many children they had. One of the women's most common complaints was that they did not produce enough milk to breastfeed their babies, followed by the question "Could the doctor please write a prescription for milk?" Women did not ask for remedies that could help increase their production of breast milk but did ask to be provided with cow's milk that they could feed to their infants instead of breast milk. Regarding these sorts of requests, the doctors and volunteers repeatedly told me— sometimes in English so the women would not understand— that the women would not give the milk to their children but would instead use it to make themselves milky chai. In a few cases, women were provided with orders for milk, but mostly they were dismissed with answers such as "There isn't any milk. We don't give out milk anymore."

Manner, dress, jewelry, bearing, education, and a host of other factors highlighted the class gulf that separated volunteers and doctors from the women and children they served. The differences in their ideas about how to maintain health and well-being were less obvious but more striking. Doctors and volunteers promoted health through particular hygiene practices and eating regimes that were beyond the practical capabilities of most women who came to the camp. Women who attended regularly were persistent in seeking health and help through their association with these powerful women who could dispense medicines and financial support. Their objectives in presenting themselves to be examined often differed from the goals of the physicians who examined them and dispensed both medical and other advice about how to live.

Even though the vast majority of the women entered the health camp shielded by some sort of burqa or other covering associated with purdah, clinical encounters put them and their children on display to one another in the waiting room and the exam room. As they sought the medical gaze for help with their problems, most women also attempted to evade it through silences, partial and mumbled answers, and averted eyes, unless crowd and circumstance compelled them to express their need more dramatically. They hesitated to admit how many children they had. Conditions of poverty made hiding reproduction desirable because they faced criticism for their high fertility—even among other Muslims—but also more difficult because they needed the camp's low-cost services. Their homes were not conducive to creating privacy, nor could they expect privacy while seeking care at the health camp or at other medical facilities. Privacy was a privilege little afforded to these mothers in daily life or in care-seeking. Millat's camp offered a space where being identifiably Muslim did not in and of itself present a barrier to treatment and so perhaps offered a better chance for a respectful medical encounter. Yet, women's adherence to religious practices—or lack thereof—could become part of clinical encounters, as volunteers and physicians made use of religious similarity to offer both counseling and criticism.

REPRODUCTIVE HEALTH CHALLENGES:
PERCEPTIONS AND EXPERIENCES

Dr. Razia

During the several months that I attended and observed the Millat health camp, Dr. Razia came regularly to see patients (*mariz dekhna*). With the style of examination that prevailed, this configuration of a medical visit reflects a fairly accurate portrayal of what took place in the examination room. Doctors looked at patients, and patients showed their bodies to the doctors (*daktar ko dikhana*). Such phrasing is not unique to low-cost health camps. In everyday speech in Hindi/Urdu, people talk about visiting a physician as "showing a doctor," a locution that echoes with the richness of South Asian notions of the power of the gaze for healing and intercession, with divinities (Eck 1998) and with doctors. I have heard endless complaints from people about the money doctors take from patients, the expensive medicines they prescribe, and the tests they order, common laments about the costs of healthcare and suspicion about the economic motives of physicians. However, patients and others also grant doctors extreme respect while in their presence, in a manner that bears striking resemblance to the ways people approach divinities, powerful patrons, and revered elders in North India.

Among Millat's physicians, Dr. Razia was the most vocal critic of patients' style of living and the most strident in giving unsolicited advice to patients. When women complained about having an insufficient supply of breast milk or of having difficulty caring for their children, she had a ready stock of responses: "Stop having children." "Take birth control pills." "Go to the government clinic and have an operation [sterilization]." She would also cite her understanding of religious perspectives and say that yes, once a fetus is conceived, aborting it is wrong, but preventing conception presents no problem.[8] When I asked her specifically about religious perspectives on managing infertility, she readily and frankly stated that God does not give children to everyone, and people facing this issue just have to learn to accept it. She further specified that one cannot take sperm or ova from someone else to get a child because Islam does not allow it.

Physicians at the health camp dismissed my queries about infertility among the patients they saw there. What they saw— here, I specify that this is what I understood to be a common perception of the doctors, not a reflection of an unconditioned reality—were women who produced too many children, some of them having babies every year, and then, because they could not care for them, bringing them to the health camp to get treatment and to beg for help in supporting them. Rehana baji responded in a more measured way and expressed more sensitivity to the difficulties facing the women Millat served. She appreciated the daily struggles they dealt with—ensuring that everyone at home had food to eat, maintaining a relatively clean living environment, and negotiating relationships with their husbands and other family members. She said, however, that while she had seen a few cases of infertility in the years she had been working with the health camp, she much more commonly saw the predicaments of women who gave birth nearly every year.

I have found it remarkable how often my questions about infertility in India, and especially about infertility among Muslim women, have led to responses that focused not on infertility but on high fertility. At times, it has seemed that people listened to me describe my research and then decided that I must have misspoken, and that I must *really* want to know about how many children Muslim women were having. This may result from their interpretation of me as an outsider who would tend to focus on high fertility in India, from their saturation in the national politics of fertility in India—which have emphasized high Muslim fertility as a problem—or possibly from not having considered infertility as a condition to be examined. The intersecting class and religious identities of women visiting the Millat camp made them likely candidates to be among the "invisible infertile," their infertility of no concern to the state or to the physicians already too occupied with the concerns of mothers and their children (Fledderjohann and Barnes 2018). On the topic of high fertility, doctors and volunteers at Millat had much to say. They cited their own personal and professional experiences; the long history of debate in India over poverty, development, and fertility rates; and campaigns by the government and by NGOs to reduce the number of births per woman. Although the goals of women attending Millat's camp and the activists conducting the camp seem to be similar—improving and maintaining health—their approaches were quite different. Women's responses to the suggestion of curtailing their fertility varied from blank stares to suppressed giggles to statements that Islam did not allow them to practice birth control. Such statements invariably led Dr. Razia to launch into lectures about how Islam did not prohibit birth control, but people did not understand the teachings of their own religion. She attributed the health problems seen among poor Muslims not to Islamic religious doctrine or practice but to their ignorance of religious doctrine and to social discrimination tied to Muslim identity in North India.

In 2006, the government of India released a highly anticipated report about the status of Muslims in India, which had been commissioned by Prime Minister Manmohan Singh. This report, now popularly known as the Sachar Committee Report (Sachar 2006) after the chairperson of the committee, has become a major reference cited by social activists as evidence for the social and economic disadvantages of Muslims in India. The report exceeds 250 pages, with nearly as many pages devoted to references, charts, and appendices. The report's task involved a particular framing of Muslims in India as a singular unit: "the Muslim community." It also required assembling data from a variety of sources, which often did not disaggregate Muslims as a single group for analysis. Given the diversity of "the Muslim community" in India, in terms of region, language, religious sect, economic class, and caste-like divisions, this project potentially required a baffling amount of data. Muslims in India, it is all too easy to forget, identify themselves not only as Muslims but also, for example, by region as Kashmiris, Punjabis, Tamilians; as members of caste-like groups—Sayyids, Pathans, Qasais; as speakers of any Indian language, such as Urdu, Bengali, Malayalam, Tamil, Kashmiri, and/or Bhojpuri; as residents of particular cities and villages; as farmers, workers, artisans, or landlords; and as men, women, or transgender people.

The Sachar committee members drew on government reports and consulted social activists working with Muslims in various parts of India. Despite critiques, the report remains a significant rhetorical tool for activists seeking to explain the living conditions of the majority of poor Indian Muslims and to advocate for change, as well as a source for further research.[9] Some of the report's conclusions help to contextualize reproductive health issues among urban Muslims as compared to other Indians. For example, the committee expressed concern about recent trends toward the concentration of Muslim population in areas they consider to be safe from unrest and discriminatory crime. The committee's concern about these settlement patterns, which they term "ghettoization," is that these areas, although considered by residents to be safe because of the religious composition of neighborhoods, often lack amenities, leading to poorer health outcomes (Sachar 2006, 14).

> The health of Muslims, especially women, is directly linked to poverty and the absence of basic services like clean drinking

water and sanitation—leading to malnutrition, anemia, a variety of diseases and poor life expectancy. . . . In some areas, higher than average incidence of TB was reported amongst Muslim women. This was partly due to the nature of their work but largely owing to poor sanitation. . . . Health services for women living in Muslim concentration areas are much worse than for women from other SRCs [socioreligious categories]. Even primary health facilities are available only at long distances. Unacceptable behavior that many Muslim women encounter at public health centres discourages them from going there. They prefer local health care providers from their own community, particularly for gynecological problems, even though they may not be as qualified. This hesitation on the part of the Muslim women to access public health facilities often leads to their ex-ploitation by private doctors. The few health care centres staffed by women doctors are concentrated in urban areas, forcing rural populations to survive with virtually no public health care. The poor quality of drinking water and sanitation in areas of Muslim concentration is another concern expressed. Population control programmes and knowledge of contraceptive practices do not reach Muslim women effectively, many felt. High rates of fertil-ity among Muslims are partly due to lack of information and the non-availability of affordable health care facilities. Besides, women often do not go to health centres which lack lady doctors. (Sachar 2006, 23–26)

The deficits identified here point to the difficulties of main-taining health in contemporary India, which are not exclusive to Muslims. However, the report's writers argue that poverty, dis-crimination, and perceptions of discrimination exacerbate risk. The chapter from which these statements are drawn focuses on public perceptions collected through conversations with Indian Muslims, including social activists, rather than on the analysis of scholarly contributions or large-scale government surveys con-ducted through various quantitative and qualitative techniques. Lack of access to basic facilities like clean drinking water contrib-ute to disease, including reproductive-tract infections (Jejeebhoy

1997, 476), among women living in poverty, regardless of religious background.

From the standpoint of fertility, the noted higher incidence of tuberculosis could contribute to infertility problems among women, should infection settle in the reproductive organs, which could damage the fallopian tubes (Bharadwaj 2001, 75; Jejeebhoy 1998, 19). Doctors often pointed to tuberculosis as one factor in infertility that sets India apart because of the high prevalence of tuberculosis in India relative to other countries. Several so-cial activists in Lucknow also often cited the poor conduct of medical professionals in government institutions toward Mus-lims as a reason why they would avoid these hospitals, despite the lower cost of care there than in the private sector. Jeffery and Jeffery (2010) also confirm the existence of such sentiments among people in rural western Uttar Pradesh (Bijnor district) with whom they have been conducting fieldwork since the early 1980s, which has been bolstered through their own experiences dealing with workers in government health facilities over many years.

Harsh treatment toward Muslim patients and subtle ways of configuring Muslims as "bad patients"—dirty, noncompliant, and difficult to deal with—were also common in clinical situa-tions in a variety of medical settings in Lucknow and are hardly isolated to health services in rural areas. Shabana baji, a social activist with whom I often had long conversations, went as far as to name a large government hospital situated in the old city—a major center of Lucknow's Muslim population—as having "com-munal" leanings that made it an unwelcoming space for Muslims. Even in the low-cost health camp run by Millat, where both doc-tors and patients were Muslim and nearly exclusively female, pa-tients tolerated harsh words and, at times, rough treatment. The construction of patients as "other" and as "bad patients," in this case, however, was based largely on class divisions, not religious ones.

Across India, examining poverty rates according to religious/caste background is itself a potentially inflammatory action, yet it is necessary for identifying and understanding existing social inequalities. The report cites the poverty rate of Muslims at 31 percent, second only to those identified as SC/ST, short for Scheduled Castes/Scheduled Tribes, castes formerly known as untouchable, and "tribes" or *adivasis* (indigenous people) for whom reservations exist in education and government employment. Among urban residents, Muslims have the highest poverty level of any category, including SC/ST, and their economic status has improved at a slower pace than that of members of other categories (Sachar 2006, 157, 161). Conditions in different areas of Lucknow are specifically referenced in the Sachar report and imply that there may be discrimination between Muslim- and non-Muslim-dominated neighborhoods in the city in terms of the provision of public services. "The study of the Muslim concentration localities of Lucknow and its adjoining areas showed a perceptible difference. . . . For instance, a Hindu dominated urban slum in Lucknow had better quality roads, drainage system, sanitation, water supply and sewage disposal compared to another slum populated largely by Muslims" (Sachar 2006, 149).

Here the categories of Muslim versus non-Muslim complicate the analysis of urban development, planning, and the provision of services. While there are surely deficits in the provision of services and infrastructure in Muslim-dominated areas of Lucknow compared to non-Muslim-dominated areas, Muslim centers of population are some of the oldest and most densely settled areas of the city and also include landmarks of historical significance that require special care in any development program.[10] Development programs in the city also often rely on the efforts of individuals to leverage their connections and influence. The relatively low representation of Muslims in government services may also play a role in these reported development gaps.

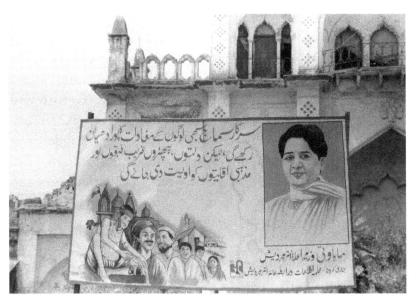

Figure 4.3. Chief Minister Mayawati's message to members of minority communities in Urdu, promising to work for all members of society, and especially members of low-caste, poor, and minority religious groups, spotted in Chauk (Chowk), the old city of Lucknow. (Photo by author.)

The Sachar report cites demographic data that show that, despite widespread perceptions that Muslims' health is distinctly worse than that of people in other communities, infant and child mortality is somewhat lower among Muslims than among members of other "SRCs" ["socioreligious categories," a term used throughout the report], but committee members express their inability to offer a conclusive explanation of this difference, which persists despite lower levels of education among women and lower economic status (Sachar 2006, 38, 237). Further research suggests that the lower levels of employment outside the home among Muslim women may contribute to these somewhat improved outcomes in terms of child death, although women's employment status has other negative impacts on their daily lives, their health, and the health of their children

(Bhalotra and van Soest 2009, cited in Wilkinson 2010).[11] Another recent paper argues that the higher use of latrines, rather than defecation in open spaces, among Muslims can explain differences in infant mortality, and that residence near other Muslims protects against disease transmission (Geruso and Spears 2015). This puzzle is far from solved. The report's writers argue that Muslims in urban areas suffer from special deprivation as compared to Muslims overall and as compared to other groups in urban areas. In addition, Muslim experiences of and widespread perceptions of bias in public-health facilities lead them to turn to private practitioners and groups like Millat for healthcare.

The women and children who attended Millat's health camp suffered from many diseases that resulted in large part from their living conditions, which included chronic problems in accessing clean water for drinking, washing clothes and dishes, bathing, and keeping their modest homes clean. Many homes had tin roofs and/or plastic bags or tarps over bamboo frames— to keep out rain, dust, and pests—that could leak or give way in adverse weather. The difficulties of escaping hot weather in the summer and cold weather in the winter also added to women's lists of health woes for themselves and their children. Even for women who conceived easily and delivered live infants with relatively few complications, there were no guarantees that their infants would survive the hardships of daily life to adulthood. Amid a seeming abundance of children hovered more stories of children lost (Pinto 2008) to life under conditions of structural violence (Farmer 1999) and of women with no children they could call their own, but few resources to get treatment or to procure children through adoption. In the *basti*, children of seven or eight might also work to help produce beautiful clothes, and those who received an outside education were often relegated to low-quality schools that promised little in terms of future advancement.

UNDERSTANDINGS OF THE NATURE OF *AULAD*:
DIFFERING DEFINITIONS, RISKY REPRODUCTION

An *aulad* is a trust (*amaanat*) of God, it's not ours. Whenever He feels like it, He will take it away.

—Shabana baji

Over the years I have attended the monthly gatherings of Shabana baji's ladies' organization, I have listened to conversations about many topics relating to women's lives, such as violence, career opportunities, religion, and politics, as well as fun and educational programs on history and literature. The meetings happen on the same date and time every month in a spacious park just steps away from a busy market in the old city. The ladies' organization is not part of Millat or Andolan, but some women who sought help from those organizations during my field research also attended these meetings. Other attendees were much more well-to-do and included prominent professionals and scholars. Although class differences were somewhat evident in women's clothing and jewelry, there was no obvious differentiation among them in terms of participation in group activities or opportunities to address the group.

Shabana baji arranged marriages and often advised women about how to deal with problems in daily life, especially disputes among family members. She allowed me to introduce my research to the members, to ask for their opinions, and to invite anyone who wished to share their experiences with me to meet later. In the same meeting, Shabana baji brought up the idea of *aulad* in a speech. As usual, the audience was composed almost exclusively of Muslim women—and no men, as a rule—from a variety of class backgrounds. She said that people generally have a misunderstanding about children—they tend to see them as their own, but this is not the case. She argued that "an *aulad* [child, progeny] is a trust (*amaanat*) of God, it's not ours.

Whenever He feels like it, He will take it away." Women who attended Millat's health camp seemed to be aware that their children could be taken away from them, as most Indian people are much more conscious about the reality of infant and child death than North Americans generally are. This is not to say that they expect their children to die and inadvertently help them on their way, as Nancy Scheper-Hughes argued was once the case in northeastern Brazil favelas (Scheper-Hughes 1992). But it is to assert that they are much more aware of the tentative nature of biological reproduction, particularly in early infancy, than people in countries with a long history of very low infant death rates.

As a woman from a wealthy, highly placed family, Shabana baji would not have been as concerned about this possibility of loss as would women living in precarious conditions with uncertain homes and income. Still, even members of the wealthiest households in India cannot completely escape illnesses resulting from periods of harsh heat and cold; contact in public spaces; travel; or pathogens carried by vendors, domestic staff, relatives, classmates, or other people in their circles of contact. Children in well-to-do households are often categorized as "weak" (kamzor) and likely to fall prey to any host of ailments, especially if they were born by cesarean section. People of all classes worry about children's health and know how quickly fevers, diarrhea, and other infections can afflict small children, though families such as Shabana baji's could be assured of the financial resources and time to care for such illnesses. Shabana baji, in this case, suggested that people tend to misunderstand the nature of their relationship with their children. In thinking that children are their "own," people feel secure, perhaps even to the extent of feeling that they own their children and can direct and command them as they please, but they forget that God can carry away their children at will—an awareness that a wealthy family like Shabana baji's could lose track of much more easily than families living in Gehumandi.

The idea of a child as a trust (*amaanat,* amānat) implies the concept of keeping-while-giving, which anthropologists working in Austronesian cultural areas have studied regarding the circulation of high-value items (Godelier 1999; Weiner 1992; Strathern 1988). In the Austronesian case, an item can be placed in circulation while the original owner retains rights in the item. The fact of its circulation does not negate the rightful owner's claim. Here, an *aulad* is more than a high-value shell necklace, but the principle is similar. God is the true owner and the rightful keeper of *aulad,* but God loans *aulad* to human parents for some unspecified period. The eventual return of the *aulad* to God is ensured, but parents tend to forget this, being caught up in their own ideas about birth, blood, and the day-to-day making of kinship that binds them to their children, as well as in the hopes of seeing the *aulad* of their *aulad.* They desire and await a grandchild, although the particular identity of the "best" child is again a matter of debate even when they wish for boys, since there are multiple options in Hindi/Urdu: *nati/natin, pota/poti*—son or daughter of one's daughter, or son or daughter of one's son—before they themselves depart earthly existence.

At the end of the ladies' organization meeting on the day I introduced my work, several women made their way to the front to offer their views in brief before heading back to their responsibilities at home. Although such encounters were a bit overwhelming, they could lead to longer conversations and inspire further questions I could ask women at my other research sites. For example, I came away with the idea that men generally hide themselves away so they can avoid blame for infertility, and their wives may shield their husbands by accepting the blame that others would so easily heap on them anyway. While problems resulting from high fertility were obvious to doctors and volunteers working with Millat, the relationships involved in managing infertility and the difficulties associated with the absence of children were less visible. As one woman in Gehumandi summed it up, "You'll find plenty of kids in Gehumandi, in the market. To some people, God has given no children, not even one. And to some people He's given children, lots and lots of children." Those many children were visible in the market and in the health camps, but the women without children rarely came to the attention of people like Millat's volunteers. Yet, when I asked members of Andolan about whether there were women in Gehumandi who had experienced infertility problems, they quickly identified two women who volunteered to share their stories with me at Andolan's office in the *basti* and a group of other residents who were willing to share their views on infertility. In the conversations we had there, I learned that the complexities of women's reproductive histories defied the neat formulations of poor Muslims and fertility that I had heard about from doctors and NGO volunteers.

Sufiya

Sufiya, a woman with no children, said that she and her husband had tried everything they could to have children, including biomedical and homeopathic treatment, but nothing helped (*koy fayda nahin hua*). Both she and her husband had been tested for every possible problem, she said, and now they had decided "to leave it up to God. If we'll have children we will, and if we won't then it's a matter of fate (*qismat*)." At the same time, she had not totally given up hope of getting a positive result by continuing to seek the help of doctors. She had gone on many fertility pilgrimages, including the famous Ajmer Sharif shrine of Sufi saint Hazrat Khawaja Moinuddin Chishti in Rajasthan, and continued to get treatment, despite her husband's objections to continuing active interventions.

> We're resting on the support of God and fate . . . my heart doesn't accept it, so I go to get treatment; I go on the sly. He [husband] yells. He says is there anything like that in God's command (*hukm*) . . . if it will happen, it will happen by just sitting around

... you're getting treatment (*ilaj*) and you're taking medicine, and you're also causing harm (*nuksan*), this and that ... even then, I don't accept it and I keep going, going on the sly to get treatment. He says, "When I don't feel tense about it, why do you? What do you have to be worried about? ... So daily work and food is in your fate, and progeny (*aulad*) are in my [someone else's] fate, why do you take it on yourself?" Even then, I go. If someone tells me [about a place], then I definitely go there, even if only one time.... I've left everything on the name of God (*allah ke naam*).

Even though Sufiya said that she was leaving it all up to God, she still felt the need to take matters into her own hands, to attempt to seek relief, an approach that the Quran also supports, as Inhorn has noted in her work on infertility treatment in Egypt (1996, 79; 1994). Sufiya's husband supported her despite their inability to have a child and over the suggestions of some of his relatives that he marry someone else, since this wife was not producing any children. As Sufiya related the story, her husband figured as something of a hero for defying his family's suggestions that he marry again. In her eyes, he was another Muslim man who cared deeply for his wife, despite criticism and any desires that he might have to obtain a child of his "own." In an ideal world, this should not seem surprising or remarkable, but it is notable because it diverges from the stereotype of the Muslim man that appears so often in media accounts of gender relations in the Muslim world that scholars feel compelled to critique and refute it (Inhorn 2006, 98).

When I asked other women in the *basti* about whether family members were likely to give women a hard time if they were unable to have children, I got very enthusiastic responses. Several women, speaking all at once, said, "If their family members don't say so, outsiders (*baahar waale*) do say so ... is there any life without children? If their children have been born early [*jaldi*, too soon after marriage, or too often], there's trouble (*museebat*);

if they've been born after a long time, there's also trouble; and if they haven't been born, there's also trouble."

Whether or not family members could be implicated, outsiders, such as people in the neighborhood, would certainly make comments about the lives of others. As these women described it, outsiders could never be pleased. No matter what happened in a woman's reproductive life—and quite possibly in her life in general—they would always have something critical to say.

It was amid this discussion about the vagaries of fertility and infertility that I first doubted whether I really understood the concept of *aulad*, particularly the gender of *aulad*. I had been repeatedly puzzled by the different ways that people interpreted and questioned my research project. Some people assumed that I must *really* be interested in high fertility rather than infertility. Others questioned whether I was *really* interested in people with no children or people with no sons. Scholarly literature and fictional representations of son preference in South Asia are vast and varied; son preference has received attention primarily in terms of ritual obligations to be fulfilled by a son, old-age economic and emotional support for parents (Vlassoff 1990), the continuity of a family lineage (Das Gupta 1987), and patterns of marriage and residence (Drèze and Murthi 2001; Jeffery and Jeffery 1997). According to the 2018 Sample Registration System Statistical Report, only 899 female children are currently being born for every 1,000 male children in India. Although Uttar Pradesh does not hold the dubious distinction of having the most imbalanced sex ratio of any Indian state, it is well below the national average, with 880 females for every 1,000 males.[12]

Both high fertility and son preference have been portrayed by the Indian government and by numerous NGOs as social problems in need of redress. Both have been the subject of aggressive media campaigns and, over time, have been approached through the provision of incentives, such as cash transfers and prizes like the now-infamous transistor radios for sterilization, and disincentives, such as ineligibility to run for local office or surrendering benefits in government jobs. The disproportionate focus on these two issues in national discourse and programs may have led people to believe that I must *really* be studying one of these two topics. The confusion, however, created an opening for me to understand the importance of the contested meanings of reproduction for women in Lucknow.

I had some sense that perhaps *aulad* bore some reference to being an heir, but I also knew that there were other words in Hindi and Urdu that specifically carried the meaning of "heir," and that are commonly used with reference to legal matters, such as the inheritance of property: *uttaraadhikaari* in Hindi and *waaris* in Urdu. I also knew the term *beaulad* (beaulād) as a common way to refer to people without children, "without-child" or childless, and heard that term used more frequently than the Sanskrit-derived *santanhin* (santānhīn), without *santan*, a term that also carries the implication of biology in a similar way to *aulad*. The term *santan* is popular enough to inspire a Hindi-language television serial that aired on the Indian channel Star Plus beginning in 2007 titled "*Santaan—Har Khushi Hai Tumse*" ("Progeny—Every Joy Is from You").

In Gehumandi, several women explained the nature of *aulad*. In the process, I also got the sense that the term might be up for debate and that some people might use definitions that suited their own circumstances or their own stances on women's rights. In this sense, the production of *aulad* is not only a physical process but also a tournament of meanings to be produced, contested, and reproduced along with children.

Q [HDS]: One question I had was, do people consider only having girls to be the same as having no child (*baccha*)? Or is there some difference?

Response: Yes, people understand it this way. Mostly people understand it this way. People say, "What are girls?"

[Second speaker]: Yes, yes, what are they? They are someone else's wealth (*paraya dhan*). You'll marry her and then she'll go to her own house [her in-laws' place].

[Munira, third speaker, a woman who had given birth to several daughters, but no sons]: Who will stay at your place? Who will help you out? I'm telling about myself. A lot of people tell me to take their son. Get it [implies property, wealth] put in my name. Why would I get it put in their name? What God approves of (*manzur hai*), that's what has to happen. If I take a boy, then are my girls no longer my *aulad*? I'll take the son of my girls. The girl [my daughter] also helps me out. My son-in-law also helps me out.

Q [HDS]: What is an *aulad*? Can any child (*baccha*) be an *aulad*, or only a boy?

Response: Only a boy. People mostly consider only a boy to be an *aulad*. They consider a girl to be someone else's wealth.

Q [HDS]: So could they say that they have no *aulad* even though they have four daughters?

Response: People say things like this. Even those who have them [girls], they say, "What do we have? We don't have an *aulad*, no one to light the lamp [no one to carry on the light of the house]." People say things like this. "When there's no boy, then who will light the lamp? Girls are outsiders."

[Munira, third speaker from above]: "Is there anyone to live in the house, who will light the lamp?" Now I'm speaking from my own place [perspective]. When I'm no longer around, my daughter will come. My daughter will light the lamp. Getting an *aulad* is essential.

Munira

Munira, the woman who had given birth to several daughters but no sons, spoke emphatically and with great conviction. She had evidently had ample opportunity to think about the issue of *aulad*. She had endured the desires of others to offer their sons to her as *aulad*, and she had rejected these offers. She redefined *aulad* to allow for the deferral of the status to the next generation, while at once asserting and discrediting the possibility of her daughters occupying the position of *aulad*. Well aware of the criticisms that others would put forth about her choices, she voiced her aspirations to procure *aulad* through her daughters. As this group of women described the views of "people" generally, boys could properly count as *aulad*, but not girls, because of their actions, which are fundamentally shaped by marriage practices in which women are expected to shift their physical residence and their allegiance to their husband's family. In this sense, girls are disqualified from fulfilling the actions idealized for an *aulad*, described here as "living in the house"—implying ancestral property and/or joint residence with parents until their deaths—and "lighting the lamp," an action that could refer to lighting up a house in the literal sense, to filling a house with life, or to continuing the family line.[13]

Munira consistently differentiated her comments between the general views of "society" and her personal views, based on her own unique life experiences. She shared her experiences with enthusiasm and conviction not only to tell her story but also to convince others of the validity argument about how people *ought* to see *aulad*. When I saw her at Andolan functions and at meetings of Shabana baji's ladies' organization, she was clearly confident in her own position and self-possessed in her work and family life. What she perceived as general social ideology differed significantly from what would serve her interests in her own life. Rather than bemoan her state as a sonless woman, she argued for social change that would give her daughters equal status as legitimate lifelong members of her household, even after marriage.

One strategy for dealing with the absence of sons among North Indian families is to recruit a *ghar jamai* (ghar jamai), a man who marries a daughter of the family and then moves into her household to take on roles that would otherwise be fulfilled by a son (Charsley 2005; Gupta 1993). The position of *ghar jamai* tends to be viewed with some suspicion and derision by people in North India. The term is usually used to criticize a man's behavior if he seems to spend too much time, effort, or resources on his wife's natal family. The *ghar jamai* role lacks prestige and can be difficult for men to fulfill, since they would be newcomers or outsiders in their wife's natal home, quite the opposite from the ideologies of kin loyalties most men are socialized into in Uttar Pradesh. As birth rates fall across India, smaller families also mean that families with an abundance of sons they would willingly redistribute to other households as *ghar jamai* may be harder to find. Munira, although a relatively poor woman living in less-than-ideal conditions, had sufficient confidence to challenge the dominant ideology in the pursuit of her own family's prosperity. She challenged the construction of an ideal *aulad* as male, yet she did not question the importance of having an *aulad* in the first place; indeed, she stated that getting an *aulad* was crucial. In the end, she wavered to some extent by saying that she would take the son of her daughters as her *aulad*—the emphasis still being on a male but on the son of her daughters (and sons-in-law), rather than of her own son. Clearly, however, being seen as someone who has successfully procured *aulad* was, for Munira, a pathway to power and respect.

RISKS IN REPRODUCTIVE JOURNEYS

At the time of my initial fieldwork, I had not yet started to think with the reproductive justice framework or to grapple with scholarship in allied-health fields that could have provided other interpretive lenses for understanding the distribution of risk in reproduction in India. Yet, grounding the rich contexts of ideologies of reproduction and healthcare-delivery encounters through anthropological literature and methods helped bring to the fore many perspectives that accord with reproductive justice approaches to research in ma-

ternal and child health. For example, listening to members of mi-
noritized and vulnerable communities most affected by health disparities and reproductive unfreedoms and paying attention to the
structural and social causes of poor health outcomes are common
aspects of research that embraces a reproductive justice approach
across disciplines.[14] While the reproductive justice framework has
been nurtured in the very specific historical and contemporary
contexts of racism and white supremacy in the United States, it also
has a great deal to offer in terms of learning to ask good questions
about and mapping the roots of discrimination that manifest in
other global contexts.

Social scientists have described infertility as a liminal state,
an in-between time and space in which those who desire parenthood also see themselves as not-yet-pregnant (Greil 1991) people
or as people caught between weak and strong identities—such
as "wife" and "mother" in the Indian context (Khare 1982). Even
people who do not suffer from infertility can continue in a liminal
state in terms of the production of an *aulad*, depending on how
they define the term, and what age *aulad* must reach before they
take the chance of considering reproduction to be ensured. Conditions of relative deprivation and high infant and child mortality
meant that these women, mostly Muslims living in the Lucknow
locality of Gehumandi, struggled to care for their families. Even
without infertility to disrupt the formation of families, successful reproduction remained far from certain. The health of infants
and small children could deteriorate rapidly due to common illnesses relating to extremes of heat and cold, poor nutrition and
sanitation, and difficulties in accessing affordable and culturally
sensitive healthcare.

The nuances of the ideal of *aulad* and the material conditions
under which reproduction happens in Uttar Pradesh raise the
stakes and the odds for women, not only because of the demands
on their own health in pregnancy, childbirth, and lactation but
also because of the risk that their children may not live long
enough to "light the lamp," and that they will be ridiculed by, and

perhaps harmed by, health workers or others along the way. Sudhir Kakar has argued in his work on the psychology of family life in India, *The Inner World*, that for Indian women taking the gamble and bearing the risks of pregnancy and childbearing, motherhood is crucial to the completion of their own personhood, regardless of their social location: "Whether her family is poor or wealthy, whatever her caste, class, or region, whether she is a fresh young bride or exhausted by many pregnancies and infancies already, an Indian woman knows that motherhood confers upon her a purpose and identity that nothing else in her culture can. Each infant borne and nurtured by her safely into childhood, especially if the child is a son, is both a certification and a redemption" (Kakar 1978, 56).

While Kakar argues for the universal Indian cultural centrality of motherhood to the constitution of female adult social identity, the costs of and risks associated with becoming mothers vary significantly depending on where in India a woman lives (especially rural or urban, north or south) (Dyson and Moore 1983) and her access to resources that promote healthy pregnancy, birth, and childrearing—factors that can, to some extent, be linked to her caste and/or religious identification (Jeffery and Jeffery 2010; Rao 2004, 151). In the years since the publication of *The Inner World*, the number of average births per woman in India has decreased steadily. Although the fertility rate varies depending on region, caste, and religion, and decreases have been uneven, family size has progressively shrunk (Jeffery and Jeffery 2002, 1997; Iyer 2002), with some regions of India now reporting fertility rates below replacement levels.[15]

Although many people in India now embrace the idea of having fewer children, preference for sons has not disappeared, a factor that has been extremely important in the use of new technologies like ultrasound for determining the sex of a fetus, followed by abortions aimed toward eliminating "excess" female children (Patel 2007b). So, the idea of each child as a "certification" and a "redemption" now needs to be qualified—unlimited fertility does not reap unlimited benefits of increased social standing for women in contemporary India. It can lead to extreme criticism from people who have embraced the small-family ideal as a key to both family and national progress, particularly if the women who give birth are from groups whose reproduction is both stigmatized and stereotyped.

Kakar's idea of safely nurturing an infant into childhood bears consideration of when a child is understood to be relatively "safe." In India, as in many other parts of the world (compare Conklin and Morgan's [1996] discussion of Amazonia and the United States), and in contrast to the contemporary practice in the United States (Layne 2003), the attribution of personhood to infants is a slow process that takes place over years. For example, in the contemporary United States, as Layne has described in great detail, fetal images become Christmas cards (and now Facebook profile pictures) and fetuses of sixteen to twenty weeks' gestation now receive names. The acquisition of new clothing, furniture, a dedicated space in the home for the new infant, and other markers of identity now commonly precede physical birth by several months. In India, across religious communities and regions, the integration of infants happens much more slowly, with common rituals of naming, giving new clothes, first haircuts, and so on, being delayed until some specified period after birth. Full personhood comes through steps that start just after birth and continue to build for years. Layne's work on pregnancy loss demonstrates the significant negative emotional consequences that can result from American expectations that a plus sign on a pregnancy test will result in a baby, and the advantages of cultural practices that advocate a more measured approach toward the process of creating new human beings.

Just how long should children be nurtured before they can be considered "safe"? The question itself highlights the liminal state of infants and their tentative status as the future of a family, a community, or a nation, and there can be no one answer, since the chances of infant survival vary so significantly depending on the physical and social locations of infants and their caretakers. That there are so many answers to this question highlights the disparities in the contemporary world that drive movements for reproductive justice. One common marker offered for the success of reproduction in North India is to see the birth of the son of one's son: a *pota*, the *aulad* of one's *aulad*. Again, the definition is open to debate, and there is no ultimate reassurance, only a series of steps toward perpetuity that continually recedes across generations. The tentative nature of fetal and infant life is lost on few people living in the Indian subcontinent, but it is further heightened for people suffering from infertility, for whom achieving even the first steps in producing an *aulad* can take on the impression of insurmountable obstacles. In a significant sense, children create their mothers in North India, and quests to become mothers take women suffering from infertility to many places in search of the completion of their identities as women and as full members of their familial and social networks.

NOTES

1. A pseudonym.

2. Clare Wilkinson-Weber's 1999 ethnography on the *chikan* industry in Lucknow provides a systematic look at the dynamics of this iconic craft production.

3. "Worth meeting," (*milne laayiq*), was a phrase people in Lucknow often used to refer me to others they thought uniquely qualified, mostly by reasons of education, class status, or their influential position, to provide insight on my topics of study. Quotes of this nature are drawn from interactions in Lucknow over the years of this study. This chapter also includes references to my fieldnotes and journal entries composed, as well as formal interactions conducted during the same time.

4. The *Indian Express* reported the yet-to-be-released census data. "Census: Hindu Share Dips Below 80%, Muslim Share Grows but Slower," 24 January 2015, http://indianexpress.com/article/india/india-others

/census-hindu-share-dips-below-80-muslim-share-grows-but-slower/. See
Jain (2015) and Pradhan (2015) on the August 2015 data release. See also
Singh (2020).

5. Census of India. Population by Religious Community, https://
censusindia.gov.in/census_data_2001/census_data_finder/c_series
/population_by_religious_communities.htm, accessed April 12, 2022.

6. A pseudonym, as are all names in this chapter. *Baji* is a general
term in Urdu that means "sister" or "elder sister" and is often used as a
term of respect. The Urdu word *Aapa* also means "elder sister" and is used
similarly to *baji*.

7. For more on Unani medicine, often known as Indo-Islamic medicine, though it connects with ancient Greek and Persian traditions, see, for
example, Alavi (2008).

8. The use of contraception, abortion, and new reproductive technologies have been extensively debated among scholars of Muslim law. There
are different interpretations of Islamic teachings among different legal
schools, on sectarian lines, and in different countries. For further reference, see Sachedina (2009), Anees (1989), and Bouhdiba (1985). In common parlance in Hindi/Urdu, the word *bacca* (child) is frequently used as
a general term, without specifying distinctions among embryo/fetus
/baby/child.

9. For example, the *New Indian Express*, June 2, 2007, says, "Counting
Heads, Missing the Picture," and argues that the report overlooks the successful artisans and craftspeople because they are outside "mainstream"
employment, such as government bureaucracy or the army. http://archive
.indianexpress.com/news/counting-heads-missing-the-picture/32470/
(Jaitly 2007), accessed September 17, 2015.

10. After the uprising of 1857 (known by many names, including the
Sepoy Mutiny), the British razed many structures in the old city, Chauk
(Chowk), to create wider roads, an action for which they received strong
criticism. Any redevelopment of these areas of the city needs to be done
with caution and sensitivity to the rights of residents. See Llewellyn-Jones
(1985).

11. The Population Reference Bureau puts the All-India infant mortality rate at 33 per 1,000 live births, compared to, for example, Afghanistan
at 50/1,000, Pakistan at 62/1,000, Nepal at 34/1,000 (all of these rates have
fallen rapidly in the last five years), contrasted with the United States at
5.7/1,000, Canada at 4.7/1,000, Cuba at 4.0/1,000, and Sweden at 1.8/1,000.
2020 World Population Data Sheet, https://interactives.prb.org/2020-wpds
/download-files/, accessed May 29, 2021. However, there is considerable

variation in the rates among regions and classes in India. Compare, for example, the 2002 rate of Kerala at 14/1,000 and Uttar Pradesh at 83/1,000 (Singh 2007). Even in Uttar Pradesh, however, the infant mortality rates appear to be dropping, with 2018 figures at 43/1,000, according to the Sample Registration System Statistical Report 2018: https://censusindia .gov.in/vital_statistics/SRS_Reports_2018.html, chap. 4, p. 137, accessed May 27, 2021.

12. Census of India. *SRS Statistical Report 2018*. https://censusindia.gov .in/vital_statistics/SRS_Reports_2018.html, chap. 3, p. 56, accessed May 27, 2021.

13. For more on the use of this metaphor by Hindu informants in Uttar Pradesh, see Khare (1982, 166).

14. For example, see Crear-Perry et al. (2021) (especially fig. 1 and discussion of the ROOTT theoretical framework, "Web of Causation: Structural and Social Determinants: Impact on Health," pp. 231–32), Chambers et al. (2021), McLemore et al. (2019), Davis (2019), and Scott, Britton, and McLemore (2019) (particularly discussion of the Black Mamas Matter Alliance's 2018 paper "Setting the Standard for Holistic Care of and for Black Women," p. 112).

15. Census of India. *SRS Statistical Report 2018*. https://censusindia.gov .in/vital_statistics/SRS_Reports_2018.html, chap. 3, accessed May 27, 2021 illustrates the trends across India.

QUIETLY PLANNING FAMILIES

Misdirecting Convention

It was a deficiency in my husband. His semen was useless. At home no one else knows that they use someone else's semen. My in-laws say to go and try somewhere else ... We thought it's possible this year we'll get some benefit, and we may not be forced to take someone else's child.

—Seema, Lucknow infertility clinic, 2007

AS I SEARCHED TO UNDERSTAND the ways that people in Lucknow, situated differently primarily by their class and religious status, moved through their relationships with reproduction as patients, physicians, advocates, and activists, I heard from them about ways of imagining kinship, motherhood, and possible ways of building families in the context of navigating fertility and infertility. People articulated their own positions and theorized about and cited evidence regarding the views of others, cultural values, and systems people might interact with, most often as the sticking points likely to present resistance or difficulty to less conventional reproduction.[1] Seema, whose story appears in more detail in chapter 2, and her husband anticipated their extended families' objections to the use of donor sperm and chose not to disclose that aspect of their infertility treatment. The prospect of clinical treatment with donor semen leading to Seema's pregnancy offered secrecy and claims to dominant reproductive ideals in ways that adoption, which they were also pondering, did not. Dr. Ahmed, who I met early in my field research, told me that she advised people suffering from infertility to consider adoption. However, she advised against adopting from within extended family networks, a strategy that interested many patients because of the interference in raising the child that would likely follow—an argument not only for secrecy but also for limiting other family ties that she saw as complicating family relationships. As part of her advocacy for parenthood, Dr. Kapoor informed people attending the prospective patient sessions at her infertility clinic that her staff could provide counseling and advice about child adoption. In each of these settings, institutions offered ways to hide the use of less-valued reproductive strategies, but some could be hidden more easily than others.

Within and beyond encounters with people in clinical spaces, I found that the contours of successful reproduction were more nuanced than having children or not having children. Munira, who gave birth to and raised several daughters but no sons, and whose arguments about gender and *aulad* are highlighted in chapter 4, took a more activist stance in defiance of social expectations about gender and family continuity. As an older low-income Muslim woman without the wealth or religious sanction to pursue a son, Munira instead drew on other cultural models, such as relying on her daughters' husbands in situations where sons came in handy. Where she could not use secrecy and with scarce financial resources to support her family, she seized visibility to argue for the roles of daughters and *their* sons to claim successful reproduction. By doing so, she neither disrupted the importance of sons nor advocated for adoption but instead temporarily turned away from patriliny to extend the possibility of family continuity through sons to future generations. People may see hiding less conventional reproductive moves as an act that upholds personal or family respectability or protects themselves or their families, but the ability to hide is stratified, and some people will defy that perceived imperative. The sparse perspectives available on adoption in South Asia suggest that disregarding discretion is more likely at the extremes, among the very wealthy or the very marginal, and this chapter focuses on the possible reasons for such actions.

In the United States, many people consider child adoption to be a default, and possibly morally superior, way of creating families, particularly in cases of infertility. In Lucknow, the topic of child adoption usually came up only if I asked about it. There are many potential explanations: the people in the middle of clinical treatment did not see adoption as an option; they saw it as something to be explored only when all other paths failed; or they saw it as an option they could not yet envision. Or perhaps they imagined it as a potential option too difficult to speak about, one that needed to be concealed because it so clearly exceeds the bounds of kinship reckoned through the bodies and bodily substances that make up dominant local versions of relatedness, especially for people who hold sufficient privilege to believe they can control reproductive outcomes. In any case, the silences, suggestions, and hints led me to look more deeply to try to understand why adoption was so difficult to follow. I was curious about what paths toward adoption might look like and what roadblocks, diversions, or roundabouts might lie ahead for people who tried to take them.

Reproductive journeys in India inevitably involve negotiations of what must be visible, and what can and ought to be made invisible, swept out of view, out of the perception of others. Women, in particular, tend to learn these arts of concealment quite early, in subtle ways that are inflected by nuances of the particular circumstances in which they come up in the world: class, caste, region, religion, the population density of their neighborhoods, the size and location of their homes, and the people with whom they share their homes. Children imbibe gendered ways of inhabiting the world through the behaviors of their elders and through the conduct required of them as they grow. In North India, children assigned to feminine categories tend to experience increasing control over their behavior, movement, and shifting forms of dress as their bodies grow, much more so than those assigned to masculine categories.

North Indian patterns of hiding women's bodies behind clothes or within walls have been well documented for decades and have been the subject of social critique and reform that has, at times, also been linked to a variety of pathologies found among women, such as vitamin deficiencies attributed to lack of sunlight created by purdah practices. The critique of social practices itself has a large scholarship behind it, from the polemical early twentieth-century *Mother India* (Mayo 1927) to postcolonial examinations of that work and its complicity in colonial rule (Sinha 2006). While purdah and practices associated with it have been thoroughly challenged from several political stances, including Indian feminist ones, various aspects of purdah continue to manifest and to be valued by a wide swath of people across genders in North India. There are a variety of practices associated with purdah, which may involve separating the sexes by creating separate spaces within homes, limiting movement outside of the home, and a variety of more and less complete ways of covering female bodies within the home or when moving outside it. These range from long tops (*kurtis*) or T-shirts to strategically placed sari ends (*pallus*) or scarves (*dupattas*) to styles of burqas that cover all exposed flesh, at times including screens that hide the eyes behind translucent fabric or shielding oneself by being accompanied by a household member. Women themselves often subscribe to such norms of modesty, endorse them, and enforce them on others, for a variety of reasons. In Lucknow, I most often heard that the times were bad, *zamaana kharab hai*, so women should dress modestly or that modest dress showed respect.

Forms of dress, especially for women, were said to reflect respect for elders or family members, professional conduct, or national pride in ways that were not just about the percentage of
skin covered—a bare midriff under a sari could complete the
requirements, while arms bared by a sleeveless blouse might
violate them. I have known many women who accepted these
expectations and conformed to them to secure permission to
move about the world outside their homes; I have also known
women who adjusted their dress depending on the audience and
venue. For example, in my hostel days, I could spot college students who were going out "Ganj-ing," to stroll in the fashionable,
upscale Hazratganj market area by the jeans and tight tops that
many of them donned, leaving behind the loose tunics and pants
(*shalwar kameez* or *churidar kameez*) that they usually wore to the
university. These students were already living away from their
natal families and could navigate their own dress with relatively
more freedom, although they still had to abide by the restrictions
of life in the university hostel, such as returning by 8:00 p.m. and
remaining inside the compound's high walls after curfew and
locked inside each dorm building through the nighttime hours.
This is another level at which women learn to—or are compelled
by others to—hide their bodies and learn the stakes of bodily inhabiting the world through daily life as they grow into adulthood.

Bodily concealments extend to the sexual and reproductive
products and desires of female bodies, and they relate to North
Indian ways of reckoning kinship. Salient metaphors include, for
example, portraying female bodies as fields that nurture male
seed (Delaney 1991; Dube 1994; Islam 1994). More and less literal interpretations of this reckoning continue to circulate and to
matter for the lives of people socialized as women, especially during their reproductive life span, from puberty to vaguely delineated menopausal older age. Strategic use of cloth, managing evidence of menstruation by hiding unused menstrual products in
paper bags and disposing of used ones discreetly, and drying

undergarments out of the sight of others are all ways that girls and women conceal tangible signs of their life stage, gender, and reproductive status. Carrying out these tasks is no small feat in crowded living spaces and inadequate housing and when menstrual products are not as accessible to low-income people, especially when clothes are dried by the sun, often outdoors. These tasks serve as beginning training for people with female bodies toward the kind of hiding intended to render sexual activity and early pregnancy invisible. Such imperatives teach that these are matters of shame (*sharm ki baaten*) that ought to be hidden from others under a literal veil of a *dupatta* or *sari pullu* that can hide undergarments while allowing them to dry or disguise a rounding belly. This level of hiding creates challenges for women's acceptance of their bodies, their sexuality, and their basic physical existence in the world. Menstruation, for example, has been a bodily state that keeps young menstruators away from school or even physically isolated in some settings. Within this system, menstruation could also provide opportunities for women to rest or take time away from work inside or outside the home.

Women's work in creating and maintaining kinship remains crucial even when its contours are not visible to all—when this work is hidden or unspoken or the credit for it is displaced to fathers who give patrilineal affiliation, priests who give names, or other men who take credit in the form of position (*kursi*, literally "seat") or power. At this historical juncture, in one way, it feels very retrograde—there are strong, vibrant feminist movements and powerful women in South Asia, after all. And yet, those movements and their demands do not filter down to the everyday lives of all women in contemporary India, or to all intimate aspects of life. There are still many girls and women who bargain for their ability to obtain schooling, to work outside the home, and to otherwise build lives of their own by acquiescing to demands from many different people, both explicit and implicit, to control their own bodies, their bodily desires, and their bodily products, the price of a measure of freedom. Remaining ignorant of, or hiding knowledge of, sex and the particular sexual aspects of women's bodies, is tied up with respectability, caste, class, and religion. Seeking to overcome infertility through biomedical treatment requires acknowledging, understanding, and working with or around these bodily realities to achieve reproduction.

Shame and hesitance around learning about or acknowledging sexuality in contemporary India are not limited to women. While the stakes are lower for people socialized as men about revealing parts of their bodies, there are still limits shaped by caste, class, and privilege. For example, in North India, being bare-chested in public has immediate associations with low-status work or living conditions. Middle-class urban men who may lounge around bare-chested in their own homes or residential colonies cringe to think of stepping outside of them that way. The prospect of a visit to a water park where men are asked to remove their shirts to enter the water can send higher-status men scampering the other way. The point here is that deeply felt historically variable social messages about the ways people ought to inhabit their bodies and the extent to which they ought to bring their physicality into the world influence how people address infertility. They demonstrate how fear of infertility is rooted not only in an absence of children but also in how people must negotiate showing up physically in the world if they acquiesce to creating, or wish to create, families that fulfill social expectations. Invisibility in reproductive processes remains a cultural ideal, one enabled by class privilege and enforced through gender norms that make it both more attainable and more desirable for some people than for others, a highly valued, but often remote, possibility.

Couples and extended families value secrecy in reproduction, yet it can be difficult to achieve, and even more so when infertility intervenes, with some strategies for alleviating childlessness offering relatively greater opportunities to maintain secrecy than others. Clinical treatment that results in pregnancy holds out the

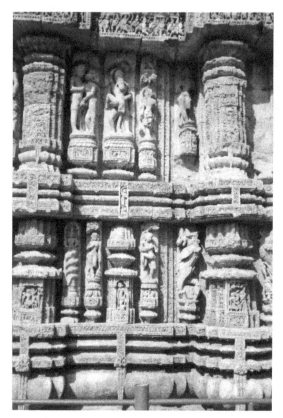

Figure 5.1. Examples of erotic art in thirteenth-century stone carvings, Konark Sun Temple, Orissa, India. (Photo by author.)

potential to keep infertility veiled from more people, and veiled in more ways, than does child adoption. Surrogate pregnancy is a more complicated issue that falls between these two extremes, and it was not, to my knowledge, a practice being undertaken in Lucknow in any of the clinics that I visited from 2005 to 2007. The use of assisted reproductive technologies (ARTs) in clinical settings can enact or approximate highly valued conception, pregnancy, and birth within a marital couple. It clearly aligns with a patrilineal logic of *aulad* imagined through the idiom of shared blood (*khun*) that permeates familial desires and messages from popular culture. Built on ideologies of motherhood and imperatives to ensure continuity of the *vansh*, a patriline, this ideal rests on privilege and is, in part, driven by fear of the results of not fulfilling desires that may be rooted beyond the body of the person who would give birth, beyond the marital couple, in the extended family. Although by no means a guarantee, the promise of *aulad* is a promise of a tie to a patriline and, more than that, of a rooting that diminishes the precarity of youth—especially the precarity of being a daughter-in-law in this system, enhancing social status, reducing the risk of being cast off. Hesitation about child adoption makes sense within this system since it does not fit this logic, and other ways of making kin garner weaker support, with the experiences of women in the roles of daughters-in-law adjusting among their marital families (*sasural waale*) serving as powerful examples. In the absence of strong alternate models of women's flourishing that seem clearly viable and attainable across classes, the threat of infertility can be a very real one. When looking across contexts of daily life, the threat manifests in multiple, stratified ways, and so do methods for evading or resolving it.

At its heart, this book is about planning families under conditions that defy the certainty and rationality that "planning" implies. These conditions of precarity, uncertainty, and loss move reproduction from planning into the realms of desire and contingency, akin to what Jan Brunson (2016) calls ever-shifting "projects of reproduction" among contemporary Nepali women. I have described some of the most intimate contexts in which people maneuver around reproductive disruption (Inhorn 2007) in search of *aulad* by using medical services, ranging from basic care at a low-cost health camp to ARTs at large biomedical facilities. People I met in Lucknow whose stories fill these pages hoped for children that could satisfy their own desires and the desires of their families and larger communities for particular kinds of people who would become the future of their families and of larger groups, whether identified by caste, religion, region, nation, language, or another relevant category. Along the way, stereotypes and disparities in risk and access to reproductive resources that structure lived experiences of reproduction in contemporary India have come into view.

Many other sorts of reproductive disruption are not part of this story but should be kept in mind. They make up part of the framing context for the stories that appear here and help make sense of why people in Lucknow searched as they did for particular sorts of children. The idea that some relationships inherently disrupt reproduction runs deep in India. Same-sex relationships that preclude marriage to an opposite-sex spouse not only threaten reproduction and impact the individuals involved; they also ripple out to larger familial and community contexts. Debates about such relationships in contemporary India are complex and are part of larger contestations with roots in (among other histories) the legacies of British colonialism. Intercaste and interreligious marriages happen, but people who marry across divisions their communities do not accept may still face ostracism and violence (Chowdhry 2007). Their fertility may be seen as disordered reproduction, creating, for example, particular challenges to finding spouses in the arranged marriage market for their children. These conflicts are surely not only about sexuality or the rights of individuals but are also about the implications of individual decisions for the present and future trajectories of larger social groups.

As the options for addressing reproductive disruption through biomedical technologies have multiplied in the world and in India over the last few decades, so have inequalities and inequities driven by economic reforms and globalization. People around the world have flocked to ARTs to attempt to solve their infertility problems, pushing other potential options for resolving childlessness, or the perceived lack of the right sort of child—a related but distinct and locally defined problem—to the wayside. In many parts of the world, child circulation through some form of temporary or permanent child fostering or adoption has a long history and falls within common, accepted, and even expected practice. Practices established during the British colonial period in India have lasting effects to the present, including legal regulations of formal child adoption that have varied according to the religious background of prospective adoptive parents. In the nineteenth century, the Rani Laxmibai, otherwise known as the Rani of Jhansi in central India, gave birth to a son who died in infancy (Jerosch 2007, 25). Just before her husband's sudden death, he adopted a child. The Rani was still a young woman. The British colonial administration refused to acknowledge the adopted child as a legitimate heir and dispossessed her of her kingdom (Jerosch 2007, 26–29; Lebra-Chapman 1986, 24–29). She became a revolutionary. A prime leader in the 1857 Rebellion, otherwise known as the Mutiny or the First War of Indian Independence, she perished in battle. She remains a potent symbol of female power, most recently reinvigorated by a long-running television serial on ZeeTV.[2] In more recent times, legal adoption of strangers, although available to some people living in India, has been a relatively rare and stigmatizing method of reproducing families.

Three major factors add complexity to the idea of adoption as a way to form families in globalizing India: secrecy; government regulation; and cultural theories of "blood," relatedness, and family cohesion. Non-Hindus and people with limited financial resources, and particularly Muslims in both categories, have been encouraged to fulfill their desire for children through means other than legal adoption in large part because of these three factors. Adoption is only one type of child circulation in South Asia; there are also various forms of fostering orphans and relatives. Although medical professionals and social workers offer adoption as a way to alleviate the suffering associated with feelings of the incompleteness of reproductive aspirations because of infertility, adopting children fails to fulfill the particular desires of many people seeking children in South Asia. The legal structure of adoption in India also makes it difficult for those wishing to bring unrelated children into their homes permanently to do so through legal means.

Aside from formal adoption, children have been transferred from their natal households to relatives' homes on a short- or long-term basis for education, most often from rural to urban areas where educational opportunities are more available and of better quality. These rural children have served as helpers in their relatives' homes—in conditions that vary from friendly and homey to exploitative—and, thus, contributed their labor in exchange for being "kept" (*rakhna*) in the household to pursue education (Karanth 2014). Relatives and nonrelatives of all religious persuasions have provided financial support for children out of a sense of obligation or charity, without creating the intimacy of formal kinship relations.

In the realm of the law, child adoption, similar to marriage, divorce, and other matters of family law, is made more complex by the history of a system that has enshrined particular interpretations of religious law, creating different possibilities depending on an individual's religious categorization (Subramanian 2014; Vatuk 2009; Williams 2006). According to British colonial-era legislation, the Guardians and Wards Act of 1890, Muslims, Christians, Jews, and Parsis—that is, persons identified as belonging to religious traditions with their origins outside of the Indian subcontinent—could not legally adopt children but could become their guardians until the child reached adulthood. A more recent secular law, the Juvenile Justice (Care and Protection of Children) Act of 2000 (JJA), which was revised in 2006, promises legal adoption without regard to the religious affiliations of adopting parents. Still, its effects on adoptive practices and cultural perceptions of child adoption are only beginning to unfold.

For example, religious law in Islam, which encompasses diverse threads of scholarship across centuries and geographies, has been interpreted as forbidding the formal adoption of children in the sense of providing them with a new name and social identity. Islamic law treats such adoption practices as a fiction and an untruth that deprives children of their rightful fathers—the relationship most emphasized—and confuses social organization (Sachedina 2009, 118, 120). These regulations severely limit the possibility of adoption for people living in countries where Islamic law influences the legal code and discourages adoption practices even outside of the formal legal framework, as Inhorn has detailed for Egypt (Inhorn 2006, 2003, 1996).

In India, interpretations of Islamic law have impacted Muslims because legal regulation of adoption, along with marriage, divorce, and inheritance, follows guidelines of Shari'a law (Desai 2009; Moosa 2009; Vatuk 2009). In Muslim families, adopting a child can have long-term effects that extend to that child's marriage. Arranged marriages within the extended family, including cousins, are possible, and marriage within larger kin networks is not uncommon. Such marriages could only take place if members of the extended family, and any religious experts they consulted for advice, accepted the child as a fully legitimate member of the family. In addition, in families that rigorously observe purdah (separation of the sexes), incorporating a person not linked by recognized biological ties or marriage into the household may require either reclassifying that person or creating new ways of managing purdah practices.

Child circulation is mentioned in scholarship on India, but it has rarely been a main focus of research, and this is particularly true of scholarship on adoption practices, with a few notable exceptions (Bhargava 2005; Billimoria 1984; Ahmad 1975). From a cross-cultural perspective, adoption and other forms of child circulation have received more thorough anthropological examination. Scholars have addressed cultural configurations of the meanings of child circulation and the potential implications for kinship (for example, Bargach [2002] on Morocco; Berman [2014] on the Marshall Islands; Bodenhorn [2000] on Inupiat in Alaska; Howell [2001] on Norway; Leinaweaver [2008, 2007] on

Peru). They have also examined governmental regulations and other factors that influence the migration of children through adoption and other forms of circulation that moved children within a single country (especially for the United States: Modell [2002, 1998, 1994]; Roberts [2002]; Strong [2001]) or transnationally (Dorow [2006]; Howell [2006]; Marre and Briggs [2009]; Volkman [2005]; Yngvesson [2010]s).

Although I did not originally intend to research adoption as part of work on reproduction, I realized during my fieldwork that ideologies about and practices of adoption could shed light on larger cultural values around family relationships. Many of my conversations in the field turned to adoption sooner or later, often because I asked whether people would consider such a step. I discussed the possibility of adopting a child with women who were undergoing infertility treatment in government clinics in Lucknow and with many women from across the social spectrum, regardless of their own reproductive status. In Lucknow, the practice of concealing adoption as a strategy for family formation seemed to continue strong. Since I focused on interviewing people who were experiencing infertility problems, I met relatively few people who had concluded their search for children through adoption—or admitted to having done so. My field data on adoption in Lucknow draws on talk about adoption by women speculating on the hypothetical possibility of someone adopting a child, by women seeking infertility treatment who might be likely to consider adoption at some point, or by medical practitioners or social workers who advised potential adoptive parents.

WANTED: DESIRABLE CHILDREN

English-language newspapers such as the *Times of India* regularly report on celebrity news from India and abroad. Several celebrities regularly turned up over the years, perhaps because of a special fascination they hold for readers and the opportunity to print revealing pictures of celebrities. News about Brad Pitt and Angelina Jolie appeared frequently throughout my stays in India from 2005 to 2011 and usually mentioned their family, which includes several children adopted from Asia and Africa and their biological children. When the family visited India for the filming of *A Mighty Heart*, news accounts speculated about "Brangelina" adopting a child from India. Indian actress and former Miss Universe (1994) Sushmita Sen has received a great deal of publicity about her status as an unmarried adoptive mother—she adopted a daughter in 2000 and another baby girl in 2010, both in India. For many Indians, these celebrities are the faces of transnational (intercountry) and domestic (in-country) adoption, although they may not name them using these categories.

Scholarly studies on adoption in India (Bhargava 2005; Bharat 1993; Billimoria 1984; Ahmad 1975) vary in their ethnographic richness and their relevance to evaluating contemporary adoption practices, since the legal regulation and administrative management of adoption has changed significantly in the last twenty years. In the limited conversations I had, I found sparse evidence of change in the "attitudes towards adoption" described in earlier works.[3] A small how-to volume called *The Penguin Guide to Adoption in India* published in 2002 reads both as an instructional manual for navigating the bureaucratic and emotional challenges involved in adopting a child in India and as an argument for normalizing adoption specifically in Indian contexts of home, schooling, and beyond.

The number of people willing and able to negotiate the legal system in India to adopt a child in-country has recently increased. Some trends in adoption practices have changed since the establishment of the Central Adoption Resource Authority (CARA), a group under the Ministry of Women and Child Development, in 1990. One of CARA's primary objectives has been to promote in-country adoption of Indian children and to oversee adoption practices and regulate intercountry adoption.[4] Whereas previously more than two-thirds of legal adoptions in India were done by foreign parents who took the child back to their home country, now the bulk of legal adoptions tracked by the CARA are in-country. Data available from the CARA indicate that the numbers of both in-country and intercountry adoptions have been declining over the last decade. In 2010, 5,693 children were placed in India and 628 abroad; for 2018–19, those numbers fall to 3,374 in India and 653 abroad, with an average over ten years of more than seven in-country adoptions for each intercountry adoption.[5] These numbers come with many caveats. They may not include in-country adoptions performed by other adoption agencies state governments in India have recognized.[6] They leave out other forms of adoption and child circulation practiced in India, including "private adoptions," which are usually organized by doctors or family-planning workers, and intrafamily adoptions, both of which happen without the legal paperwork required for a formal adoption. The listing of numbers reveals little about how adoption gets represented by adoptive parents to the children involved or to their wider circle of family, friends, and neighbors.

Vinita Bhargava (2005) has provided a particularly rich account of adoption in India, describing efforts by more recent governments to standardize and legalize adoption proceedings and providing a window into the experiences of Indians who have adopted children through the legal system, using adoption agencies. Bhargava was the parent of a biological son and an adopted daughter, as well as an executive member of an adoption advisory committee. In New Delhi, India's capital city and the main center for in-country legal adoptions in North India, she conducted interviews with adoptive parents and adopted children (2005, 12, 14–15, 31). Her study identified infertility as one of the main motivations for adoption in India. She carefully points out the limitations of the scope of her study, including not only the form of adoption but also the generally high class, caste, and educational levels of adoptive families participating in the study. Recent demographic scholarship based on research in South India points to the possibility that less privileged families may be more likely to opt for informal adoptive strategies (Unisa, Pujari, and Ganguly 2012). Still, Bhargava's study provides a valuable complement to work that examines adoption from the point of view of couples undergoing treatment in biomedical infertility clinics.

For nearly all of the women I interviewed in clinics in Lucknow, adoption seemed to be a remote possibility, a hypothetical course of action that they might or might not consider in the future. Most of them reserved adoption as an option only in case they truly lost hope about the possibility of conceiving a child, a view of adoption that accords with what Anjali Widge (2005, 230) and Aditya Bharadwaj (2001, 2003) found in their interviews with people being treated in infertility clinics in New Delhi, Mumbai, and other large cities. Only a few people I met brought up adoption on their own as an option they might pursue. Among women undergoing treatment in infertility clinics, just one very frankly volunteered that she had already registered with an adoption agency and said that she and her husband were very serious about adopting a child, even though they were continuing to try to conceive with the help of biomedicine.

Several physicians I interviewed advocated for the adoption of unknown children from organized agencies, yet they said that most people who sought their advice preferred the idea of adopting a child from within their own extended families. Physicians emphasized how, from their point of view, the difficulty of dealing with other claimants to a child's affection and care mattered more than concerns about taking in a child of unknown origins. In adoptions within families, as one gynecologist pointed out to me, other family members would be likely to interfere with the child's upbringing and to criticize the care given by the adoptive parents, with comments such as "He's become so thin" (*dublapatla*), which implies that no one looked after his welfare or fed him properly. Rather than being a compliment, as some people raised with cultural associations of thinness with health, wealth, and beauty might assume, in this context it's usually a critique of someone's living situation—students away from home at university, living in a hostel with poor food and no one to look after them, or people working too much and neglecting proper meals and rest. Physicians gave their perspectives to patients asking for advice: a child's known origins within the family would be an attraction for adoptive parents but would also present an obstacle to successfully shifting the child from one part of the family to another.

In a frank discussion about her work in the government family-planning program, Mrs. Farooqui,[7] a retired counselor, spoke with me about childless couples who came to her for advice about how to plan their families, often begging her to find an infant for them to adopt. She confirmed many of the stories that Bhargava notes as being part of the popular lore about methods of going about adoption, but she did not find these to be borne out in her research with families in Delhi (Bhargava 2005, 69, 93). In Lucknow, Mrs. Farooqui told me that she had seen women simulating pregnancy by tying pillows around their stomachs, which gradually expanded until the time of their "delivery," by which time they hoped Mrs. Farooqui would have found a suitable match for them. She reported that some women claimed that they kept their husbands unaware of this act by saying that their doctor had strictly forbidden their husbands from touching them until the baby's birth. Such simulations might conclude with frantic calls from women saying something like "I'm in my tenth month now . . . will you have a baby for me soon?"

The matches that Mrs. Farooqui said she helped to arrange fall into a category she identified as "private adoptions." New parents who wanted to give up an unwanted baby—usually a girl, often because of the number of children already at home, were matched with a childless couple within the confines of a hospital and without paperwork. In most cases, Mrs. Farooqui argued, both those giving and receiving the child preferred not to leave a paper trail to maintain secrecy. She could not recall a single family that had openly adopted a child in this manner. The CARA has been working to prevent "private adoptions" because of their potential to lead to abuse, child trafficking, and coercion of birth parents who could later change their minds about abandoning a child. The CARA website, guidelines for adoption issued in the *Gazette of India* dated July 2015, and the *Penguin Guide* all specifically mention adoptions of this sort to dissuade prospective adoptive parents from attempting one (*Gazette of India* 2015; Lobo and Vasudevan 2002).

Mrs. Farooqui said that she suspected that her assistant took money on the sly for helping childless couples obtain children through private adoptions. When I later spoke with her former assistant separately, she intimated that Mrs. Farooqui may have taken money from childless couples. I had no independent confirmation of money changing hands. Both of these women struck me as committed and genuine advocates for families— including their own—who had been deeply immersed in their position as government servants. Such insinuations, true or not, would not surprise people accustomed to dealing with Indian bureaucracy. Corruption through demands for and provision of cash, favors, and *mithai* (sweets) is well documented (Gupta 2012; Jauregui 2014), and people generally expect that getting their matter resolved through government offices will require finding and "obliging" the right person with the right amount, whether or not an official actually demands a bribe. Suggesting that someone else in the office or hierarchy engages in such practices can be a way of claiming innocence for oneself.

Part of the appeal of a private adoption is the chance to adopt a newborn, which adoptive parents can more easily present as their biological child. Mrs. Farooqui reflected that, in her experience, people were quite anxious to have a child of their own "blood" (*khun*), but if this was not possible, they would consider a private adoption, taking the opportunity to maintain secrecy about adoption and to fully experience *mamta*, motherly affection. Interference by biological parents could otherwise inhibit *mamta*, especially in the case of adoption within extended families. Many couples tried to find out from her the origins of the child with whom they would be matched. Muslims, in particular, questioned her about the source of the *nutfa*—literally "semen" or "sperm"—involved in creating the child, with relatively few worries about the origins of the ovum or of the woman who gave birth to the child.

According to Mrs. Farooqui, some Hindus and Muslims tried to find out about the religious identification of the baby to be adopted, although she would try her best to convince them that the child's origins did not matter, telling them, "So many Sitas have gone to Maryam's place, so many Maryams have gone to Sita's place." Sita is a common Hindu name, and Maryam is a common Muslim name, both for girls, with their own cultural references—Sita, a goddess and wife to Lord Rama; Maryam, mother of the Prophet Isa (Jesus). Her statement emphasizes the interchangeability of infants in terms of religion and the prevalence of girl babies in such adoptions, while according an exalted position to infants their parents decided not to keep. Mrs. Farooqui's former assistant also seconded this sentiment, saying that "children have no caste [*jat*]." While others working in Uttar Pradesh have also recorded similar ideas, implying that children acquire their caste status primarily through consumption rather than through birth (Pinto 2008, 262), people considering adoption do express views that even an infant is not a blank slate, because every child comes from somewhere, and that background, they say, will influence the development of the child and the match between child and household.

After completing a private adoption, Mrs. Farooqui explained to me, adoptive parents could quite easily go to the government office that issues birth certificates and state that their baby was delivered at home, which would explain why there was no documentation of the baby's birth from a hospital. At that time, half of all births in India still took place at home,[8] so such a strategy may not be blatantly absurd. However, for the middle- to upper-class urban people who most often adopt children, delivery at home is now quite unusual. Within government bureaucracy in India, many unusual things have been made to happen by paying the correct fee to the correct official, thereby earning adoptive parents a birth certificate that carries their names, which could later be used to prove their parental identity and the child's age for school admission. Mrs. Farooqui's former assistant told me about this issue and said that husbands and wives would arrange to have the birth documented as a home delivery with them listed as the birth parents. Usually, there would be no inquiry about their claims through a home visit from the police (standard practice for other applications, such as for a passport or a formal, legal adoption), and certainly no medical examination of the woman identified as the mother. Bhargava says that at the time of her study, the fee required for the issuance of such a certificate was around 1,000 rupees (approximately 25USD), an appreciable cost even for middle-class parents, but not expensive enough to be prohibitive.

UNDERCOVER MORAL PIONEERS?
PURSUING CHILDREN IN SECRET

Almost every woman I met seeking infertility treatment in biomedical clinics in Lucknow in 2007 claimed to be keeping some aspect of her and her husband's treatment secret from someone. However, the level of secrecy and the degree to which others were excluded from knowledge or informed in order to seek their assistance in facilitating treatment varied. Some women said that their in-laws knew they were seeing doctors but did not know the particulars of their treatment. Others were more careful to keep their treatment secret from people in their natal home (*maika*) to save their family members from what they saw as unnecessary worry. The prospects for maintaining secrecy in adoption are much more dubious than in seeking children through the use of ARTs, which serves to promote the services of clinics offering these technologies and to encourage people suffering from infertility to put off considering adoption as a way of fulfilling their child desire.

The secrecy evident in both of these types of reproductive pursuits in Lucknow suggests a deep sense of discomfort among prospective parents about publicly deviating from the standard conventions of childbirth and of becoming "moral pioneers" (Rapp 1999) to create Indian families that, despite being heteronormative, openly defy the link between marriage and procreation. Bharadwaj argues that "an adopted child breaks the link between the body and the progeny and becomes a visible 'third party' in a way that makes it impossible for family groups to collude in a conspiracy of silence" (2003, 1875). The kinds of adoptions that Mrs. Farooqui could help arrange have the potential to preserve this link, albeit through some measure of deception and creativity, while the adoptions offered legally by the government offer a greater threat of severing it. However, private adoptions also suffer from a high potential for abuse, possibly shading into child trafficking (Lobo and Vasudevan 2002). Here, much depends on the honesty and goodwill of the individuals involved in handling each case, whereas the legal system theoretically avoids those problems by creating standard procedures for evaluating adoptive families, their background, and their home environment. With the dubious regard many Indians have for government bureaucracy, however, legal procedures are far from unblemished, while private transactions get their legitimacy through the reputations of the individuals involved. In this sense, the trust and faith involved resemble those expressed by villagers in Pinto's work on medical practitioners in rural Uttar Pradesh. Villagers favored the local *kaccha* (raw/without formal training)

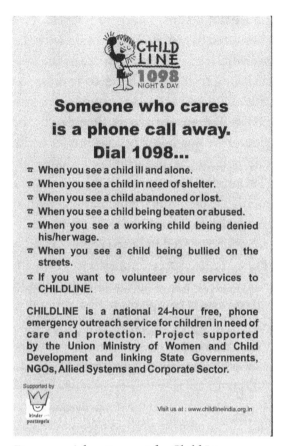

Figure 5.2. Advertisement for Child Line, opposite sides printed in English and Hindi.

doctors, whose family backgrounds they knew and respected and
with whom they were embedded in local webs of relationships,
over practitioners in government facilities, who tended to ridicule
them on the rare occasions they made themselves available for
consultation (2004). Personal connections and local links may
matter more than formal credentials or official standing.

Although CARA advises legal adoption centers to counsel prospective adoptive parents about the importance of revealing the
details of adoption to children at an age when they are prepared

to understand what it means, Bhargava notes that many parents in her study hesitated to talk about adoption with their children. Many of those who refused to participate in the study gave this reason for declining to meet with her to express their perspectives (2005, 138). Desires to maintain secrecy may center on the child, the extended family, people in the neighborhood, and/or society in general. While adoptive parents in India have been shown to focus more on the importance of "doing" kinship rather than "being" kin (as in McKinnon 2005, 115), many of them shy away from openly proclaiming their creation of kinship ties with children through the paperwork of legal adoption.

Women in Lucknow cited concerns about an adopted child's ability to "adjust" to their new homes. However, in contrast to Bharadwaj's interlocutors in large Indian cities (2003, 1877), they rarely referred to genetic composition to express doubts about a child's origins or ability to adjust. *Khun* ("blood") was a much more commonly cited factor for thinking about adjustment in an adoptive household; however, the sentiments expressed are similar. "Inherited qualities," whether expressed through the idiom of genes, blood, the traces of actions in previous lives (karma), or in general, took on an almost mythic sheen in the view of many informants, as if they were mysteries contained within an individual, just awaiting their time to be revealed.

If *khun* is the overriding concern of an individual, couple, or their extended family members, then the adoption of a stranger does not guarantee a solution to their desire for children, and even adopting within the extended family may only provide a partial answer. If, on the other hand, gaining an opportunity to experience *mamta* or to raise a child is the central concern, then adopting an unrelated child through legal channels provides one possible solution. However, this option historically has not been equally available to all Indians. Legal regulations based on the religious identification of the people wishing to adopt and the tendencies of people working in adoption centers to eliminate some prospective parents from consideration because of their class background, religious identification, or other idiosyncratic factors, have placed limits on adoption as a potential reproductive option.

WHY NOT ADOPT? LIMITS OF THE LAW FOR
FULFILLING REPRODUCTIVE DESIRES

With the blessings of elders we got married in June 2002. Both of us are from middle class south Indian families. As it would be, we were a happily married couple. After few years of marriage, when my wife did not conceive, we consulted few fertility experts in Bangalore. We spent a fortune on procedures, which resulted in nothing but pain, suffering, huge body changes due to artificial injections of hormones and financial loss. Then we decided enough is enough. We thought why we don't adopt a baby.

—C. J. Bharath and S. B. Mandakini[9]

For people seeking to adopt children through legal channels in India, the path to parenthood through adoption is far from simple. This couple successfully adopted a daughter through an agency, according to the short account on the CARA website. However, important differences emerge in the ability of willing adoptive parents to obtain a child, based primarily on class and religion. Until recently, there was no uniform code under which all Indians could legally adopt a child. Under the Hindu Adoptions and Maintenance Act of 1956 (HAMA), Hindus, Buddhists, Jains, and Sikhs may legally adopt a child. However, the HAMA has limitations—people with a biological child or children may only adopt a child of the sex that is not represented among their biological children. So, a person with a biological daughter could only adopt a son, and vice versa (Lobo and Vasudevan 2002, 26).

The provisions of the HAMA are available for people whose religious traditions originated in South Asia, whether they belong to that group through birth or conversion. Children adopted under the HAMA receive a legal status equivalent to US versions of legal adoption, including inheritance. The JJA of 2000, revised in 2006, offers people who would otherwise adopt children under the provisions of the HAMA a chance to avoid some of the limitations imposed by the HAMA. A judgment rendered in 2009 by Judge D. Y. Chandrachud of the Bombay High Court clarifies the nature of the JJA and raises significant questions for the implications of this law for the previously existing personal laws, especially the HAMA and the Guardians and Wards Act of 1890 (GAWA). In this case, a couple with a living biological daughter wished to adopt a girl child, which would not have been permitted under the HAMA's provisions. The judge pointed out that the JJA is a secular law intended to handle a general social issue of dealing with abandoned and orphaned children. "The Hindu Adoptions and Maintenance Act, 1956 and the Juvenile Justice Act, 2000 must be harmoniously construed. . . . While enacting the Juvenile Justice Act, 2000 the legislature has taken care to ensure that its provisions are secular in character and that the benefit of adoption is not restricted to any religious or social group. . . . The human tragedies of orphaned and abandoned children straddle social and religious identity. The urge to adopt is a sensitive expression of the human personality. That urge again is not constricted by religious identity"[10] (Chandrachud 2009).

The petitioning couple was granted permission to take advantage of a secular law to override the strictures of law based on religious identification. The judge expressed sensitivity toward the difficulty of balancing the new, secular, and universal JJA with the existing personal laws. In India, family issues such as marriage, divorce, adoption, and inheritance—referred to as "personal law"—are governed according to the religious laws of different religious groups, rather than applying a single universal code to all Indian citizens. By citing the suffering of children available for legal adoption, the judge attempted to sidestep the controversy involved in allowing people to adopt regardless of the religious restrictions, effectively endorsing a universal code. According to the *Indian Express*, this same rationale was used to allow Sushmita Sen to adopt a second daughter. Sen adopted the first, Renee, under the HAMA, and the second, Alisah, under the newer JJA. "Today, after Justice V M Kanade [in Mumbai] allowed Sen's adoption petition, Sen said, 'Adoption is about reverence, it's not charity. More and more people should come forward to adopt. We believe in ties of the heart, not just those of blood. I will adopt as many children as I can raise.'"[11]

Here, Sen strategically placed herself as a spokesperson for parents who have adopted children and argued for a theory of relatedness that legitimizes her own family and acknowledges the mainstream beliefs against which she has taken a stand by adopting unrelated children. She has repeatedly made such statements about her status as a mother and has spoken to the media about the challenges she faced in adopting as a single woman. In terms of religion, after a gap of ten years, she was able to navigate around legal restrictions to adopt a second daughter.

Muslims, Christians, Jews, and Parsis, whose religions are identified as originating outside of the Indian subcontinent, were not able to adopt children under the HAMA but could become the legal guardians of a child through the GAWA. Children adopted under this act are entitled to only limited rights, which end when the child reaches eighteen. The JJA offers a way for people belonging to these religious groups to adopt a child and give them equal rights and status as children adopted through the HAMA. The ways the JJA will be applied and interpreted are still being tested as cases come before the courts.

In 2007, the *Times of India* reported on a legal case filed by a prominent Muslim couple with a biological son who had adopted a daughter under the GAWA. The mother, Shabnam Hashmi, petitioned the Supreme Court in 2005 for uniform adoption rules. According to the news, her move was prompted by several instances when their daughter was denied benefits because she was not legally a full member of their family (Mishra 2007, 1). The All India Muslim Personal Law Board (AIMPLB) strongly opposed the provision of full adoption for Muslims under Indian law. Since Islamic law as interpreted in India does not permit full adoption, Indian law has also upheld this restriction for Muslims in India. Any move to create a uniform law for all Indians in matters of personal law has provoked strong reactions from Muslim clerics and other authorities who claim to defend minority rights. There are often disputes among Muslims about who should represent their voices, particularly between men and women, whose interests can be strongly at odds with each other, while formal religious leadership is nearly exclusively male.[12] Hashmi and her husband, Gauhar Raza, argued that they should be able to adopt a child without being compelled to bring their religious identity into the picture. She responded to the criticism of their petition by the AIMPLB, saying, "I am not at all advocating that adoption laws should be forced on Muslims. But those who want should be given the freedom to bring a baby home without any fuss. Unfortunately, at the moment it is easier for a foreigner than a Muslim to adopt a child in India" (Mishra 2007, 6).

Muslims wishing to adopt a child were obliged to approach the state apparatus not simply as citizens but *as Muslims*. Hashmi and Raza adopted their daughter, who was twelve at the time the case appeared in the national press, through the GAWA and before the 2006 amendment to the JJA of 2000, which specifically addressed adoption (Gogoi 2014, 4). An editorial that appeared in the *Times of India* to comment on the state of adoption laws in India was preceded by the caption "A Thought for Today." The thought for the day was, appropriately, a quote from Rabindranath Tagore, one of India's most famous nineteenth-century writers: "I shall be called by a new name, embraced by a fresh pair of arms" (*Times of India*, November 12, 2007, 10). In terms of Islamic law, there is no problem with an abandoned child being embraced by a new family. The main difficulty lies precisely in the attempt to change a person's identity based on the lineage of the biological father (*nasab*) by giving him or her a new name and a new network of kin relations, while stripping him or her of relationships based on his or her paternity. Sachedina (2009) has examined this issue extensively in his work on Islamic biomedical ethics: "'He has not made your adopted sons your sons in fact. Call them after their true fathers. That is more equitable in the sight of God' (33: 4–5) ... biological parents remain the legal parents, and the guardian fulfils the obligations to the child in substitution for the biological parents" (2009, 118, 120).

The basics outlined here have applied to the regulation of adoption among Muslims in India, although there is room for variation among various schools of Islamic law and the judgments of particular Islamic scholars. Sachedina is clear that the major disputes regarding the terms of full legal adoption and the use of particular reproductive technologies revolve around concerns about the confusion over a child's heritage, and above all about paternity, so that adoptive motherhood remains largely left aside. I heard similar sentiments echoed by some prominent Muslim activists in Lucknow.

In my interactions with people suffering from infertility, many Muslims bracketed the opinions of Islamic scholars from their explorations of their options to get children, and Hindus rarely consulted any religious authority, although people from both communities might seek divine intervention by visiting shrines (*dargahs* or *mazaars* in particular) or temples. Both Hindus and Muslims who were actively engaged in biomedical infertility treatment said that their problem was one rooted in the body and for which they needed the intervention of doctors, not religious experts. Many reform-minded Muslims in Lucknow asserted their desire to conduct their daily lives without the intervention of religious authorities. However, regarding "personal laws," they had limited options for escaping the control of religious law, whether or not they agreed with the interpretations of Islamic law that have been enshrined in the Indian legal code, which is itself largely an artifact of the period of British rule. The law has accommodated religious diversity among citizens, but it has also compelled citizens to approach the state according to these categorizations. Authorities on Islamic law in India have often opposed legal actions that attempt to change the legal structure (Baird 2005; Bajpai 2011; Cuno and Desai 2009; Rajan 2003; Subramanian 2014).

Recent rulings on child adoption in India have sought to move away from legal divisions based on religious identification, which judges have noted in their rulings, from Judge Chandrachud in the 2009 case mentioned above, to Judge Ranjan Gogoi and colleagues in their 2014 ruling on Shabnam Hashmi's case. Ruling in favor of the right of Muslims, or Indians belonging to any religious group, to legally adopt a child under the JJA (United News of India 2014), Gogoi asserted that prospective parents could choose to work through laws created with their religious identity in mind or through the universal code, setting religious guidelines aside (2014, 9).

The judge wrote at length about the legislation as a "small step" toward a uniform civil code, a legal code that would apply equally to all citizens of India. Support or opposition to this legislation might rest not on ideas about the best interests of a child to be placed for adoption but on support for or opposition to a uniform civil code. Such legal and political complications provide incentives for prospective adoptive parents to act quietly whenever possible.

Rehana baji, a prominent social activist in Lucknow and one of the main volunteers at Millat's health camp (see chapter 4), described a case in which she helped to arrange an adoption. She had been approached by a couple who lived abroad and planned to take the child with them. The couple who adopted the child gave a gift of 50,000 thousand rupees (about 1100USD) as compensation to the family that gave up their daughter, but Rehana baji did not describe this act as a form of selling the child or as a form of exploitation. In reflecting on this case, Rehana baji said that the biological mother of the child later came to ask about how the girl was doing. Rehana baji assured her that she was fine but did not provide her with any way of establishing contact with the girl because she was concerned that the adoptive family be protected from the threat of blackmail. However, she said she did not feel good about the whole thing. In accordance with Islamic law, she supported people taking in children to facilitate children's care. Still, she cited a version of Islamic guidance, saying that "a son does not become a son by making him so, nor a daughter. It's a blood relationship (*khun ka rishta*)."[13]

The experience left Rehana baji feeling uncomfortable, especially about the child being separated from her birth family. With great sadness in her eyes, she quoted a couplet (*sher*) from nineteenth-century Urdu poet Ghalib. The language of Ghalib's poetry is notoriously difficult to interpret, not only because of the range of vocabulary but also because part of the art of the *sher* is to create a multiplicity of possible meanings using only two lines. I appreciated the sounds of this couplet but could not grasp the larger meaning, something that people who are very well versed in literary Urdu often expect from others who are less thoroughly grounded in the tradition, including many contemporary Indians. The couplet was meant to communicate the idea that when people get used to worries, they start to seem easy, a sentiment Rehana baji echoed in her social-work pursuits and descriptions of her experiences with her late husband's illness and death.

The ambivalence that Rehana baji felt about adoption is emblematic of the dubious cultural legitimacy attached to permanently relocating children from one household to another in North India, particularly among Muslims. I have heard many people comment on highly publicized adoption cases and blended biological families with a mixture of disbelief and respect for those parents' openness to taking on the responsibility of raising "someone else's" child. Cultural values about how families can and should be created play into decisions about whether to adopt and, if so, how to adopt. These values may be inflected by a family's background, and government regulations have historically stratified the possibility of adoption, with adoption rights depending on religious identity. For people who attempt to take the culturally daring step of adopting an unrelated child, perceptions of the leverage and discretion exerted by particular officials in particular adoption centers to accept, reject, accelerate, or delay a couple's application support the idea that access to legal adoption is also stratified.

Based on the existing legal framework, access to the formal system has not been equal. Bhargava (2005, 48) found that in some adoption agencies, Hindus were considered prospective parents, while people identified as belonging to other religious backgrounds were turned away because the children would be given unequal legal rights, making Hindus by default the most desirable adoptive parents. Applicants with more education and higher incomes were often assumed to be better candidates than those with fewer resources. Whether or not the JJA eliminates or minimizes this dynamic remains to be seen, based on how the JJA will be harmonized with other adoption laws, but also on how legal change affects the many small decisions adoption professionals make to match children with parents.

In Bhargava's work, some agencies requested or required applicants to submit doctors' reports attesting to the couple's infertility problems, which deterred people not suffering from infertility from applying. Although the CARA issued guidelines for adoption agencies in 2004 in an attempt to regularize their practices, even in 2006–07, I found evidence that agencies preferred infertile and relatively wealthy applicants to others. Workers I spoke with in Lucknow talked about the relative paucity of children available for adoption as a major factor in screening applicants, as if there should be a triage system for the distribution of children.

Most of the in-country legal adoptions in India have historically taken place in a few urban centers. There are more children available for adoption than are getting placed in-country. The CARA regulations set out specific steps to try to place children locally before they can be offered for inter-country adoption. With hundreds of children being given in inter-country adoptions each year even in recent times, there appears to be a gap between the children that are available for adoption in India and the desires of Indians adopting children. Bhargava (2005) has argued that one part of this gap may be linked to administrative difficulties, including problems in transferring children from one state to another within India and allegations that adoption workers eager to facilitate inter-country adoption take steps to discourage Indian applicants from accepting certain children, clearing the way for them to be sent abroad. Aside from these sorts of issues, the desire for a particular sort of child—male or female, with a certain skin tone, in good health, of the right age—also leads to the creation of categories of children who either remain in adoption centers or get placed with families settled outside of India.

In Lucknow in 2007, adoption workers compared the process of placing children in adoptive homes to a father searching for a husband for his daughter. Just as a father does everything in his power to arrange a marriage—a new home—for his daughter with the best sort of man, so do agency employees look for the best parents for the children under their care. Income was clearly part of gaining an endorsement as "best parents." On separate visits, workers cited to me a minimum monthly income of 5,000 or 7,000 rupees (at the time, 110/155USD, a lower-middle-class salary) as the minimum for adoption—a requirement that might be overlooked if the applicants could show equivalent resources in property, such as agricultural land. They said that people looking to adopt children most often preferred boys, and that they also looked for newborns. In this center, there were roughly equal numbers of boys and girls, but girls had more often been abandoned as newborns, while boys were generally older children who had run away from home. In a single year (2010) in Lucknow, by September, 20 abandoned children had been recovered, out of which 16 were girls (2008: 17 girls out of 24, 2007: 19 girls out of 21) (*Times of India*, September 2, 2010).

On my first visit to a large adoption center in Lucknow, I spoke with one of the government employees in charge of the agency, who cited facts and figures about adoption and gave me copies of the relevant legal documents. On another visit, I talked mostly with several young men, university students who worked part-time with an organization that rescues lost, abandoned, and abused children that operated out of the same center. These workers were more poetic in their evaluation of the work done by people in the agency to match children with particular homes. They said that they search for families that can make the child into a good citizen (*naagrik*) because otherwise, the government could just keep the responsibility of raising the children, rather than placing them in homes where they might not get good care. They suggested that poor families might have bad intentions and adopt many children, then force them to beg to increase their income. These students' prejudices about the potential for poor families to be "good parents" according to their own expectations were evident. Couples with no children got first preference, they said, because they would be able to love an adopted child the best, and without that, the parents would discriminate between their biological and adopted children.

All of these workers focused on finding the right families for the children under their care, whereas what I had seen from the perspective of infertile couples was a focus on finding the right children for the families that desired them. Bhargava cites the idea of moving from thinking of adoption as "families for children" to "children for families" as one of the main controversies behind inter-country adoption (2005, 27), one in which the dynamics of adoption shift based on one's perspective and on the match or mismatch between the availability of children in need of homes and people searching for children to bring into their homes. The evaluation of the home environment by agency workers and assessments of income, fertility status, and the general manner of prospective adoptive parents leaves workers plenty of room to make their own judgments. Whether or not they occur in practice, popular perceptions about government bureaucracy influence how members of the public and prospective adoptive parents think about adoption. These perceptions include ideas that employees in adoption agencies may be swayed by their own preferences and prejudices in evaluating applicants' suitability as parents, and that in some cases extra cash may change hands, none of which helps to destigmatize legal adoption.

In July 2015, the CARA released newly revised and updated guidelines for adoption in Hindi and English[14] that set out proper procedures for adoption. These include a multitude of forms to be completed during proceedings, standard questions for home studies and other parts of the process, clear guidance about the fees and documents required, and the order of preference for prospective adoptive parents. The hierarchy outlined gave priority to domestic adoptive parents and then to Indian citizens residing outside of India, and decreasing preference to other people with more tenuous or no connection to India. Although the guidelines include a long list of documents required to complete an adoption, Schedule 8 concludes with a note that stands out as conflicting with, and perhaps responding to, popular ideas about who might consider adopting a child. It reads, "NOTE: Infertility certificate is NOT required for adoption." (*Gazette of India*, July 17, 2015, 105).

THE EFFECTS OF "BLOOD" (*KHUN*): WORRIES ABOUT HOW THIEVES, ROBBERS, AND RESPECTABLE PEOPLE ARE MADE

Among women suffering from infertility who talked with me about the possibility of adoption, none said that they had actually adopted a child. Whether or not they were considering

adoption for themselves, they commented on several difficulties they feared they would encounter if someone brought an
unrelated child into the household. First, they doubted whether
their other family members would accept the child. They wondered about how the child's loyalties would develop as they grew
older and about the psychological effects of adoption on the
child. They were skeptical about whether an adopted child would
be able to "adjust" in their families. The concept of adjustment
usually described relied not only on the development of inter-
personal relationships but also on cultural theories of relatedness,
harmony, and "fit" within the household.

What is at stake in cases of adoption in Lucknow, and particularly in cases of adopting strangers, is similar to the danger and
difficulty people in North India tend to associate with bringing
new members into a joint household through marriage. However,
it is not precisely the same because infants and very small children, those most likely to be adopted, do not come with long-held
sets of habits, preferences, and expectations that create challenges
to incorporating new daughters-in-law into the household or of
developing bonds between children and a father's new wife. *Sauteli mas*, or stepmothers—women who marry a child's father after
the death of or divorce from a previous wife, or as co-wives—are
typically labeled as "bad mothers" because of their lack of blood
relation with the children placed under their care. Relations defined through shared "blood" (*khun*) are portrayed as more stable
than other relations. Still, they also come with their own dangers,
many of which involve the very division of loyalties, affection,
and property that are often cited as reasons for not incorporating
new members into a family through adoption.

Women fretted to me about the impact that adopted children's
blood (*khun*)—and, implicitly, undesirable inborn traits likely to
accompany the child's unknown caste and religious origins—
might have on their ability to fit into an adoptive home and to develop affection toward members of the adopted family. Adopting

a child from within the extended family; that is, from within a woman's *sasural*—from among her husband's relatives—would alleviate these worries about *khun*, making adoption more acceptable. However, it would also shift the balance of inheritance for any family property, potentially creating new areas of alliance and/or competition within the extended family. Many people also commented that neighbors and others who knew about the adopted status of a child would make it difficult to raise that child because they would tell the child the "facts" about their origins and generally create problems, regardless of the child's origins within or outside of the extended family. In Muslim families that still form marriages within relatively close degrees of relationship, the idea of integrating an unrelated child into the household is farther still from the norm, since even new daughters-in-law can come from within the larger family group.

    Khun served as a major idiom through which people in Lucknow articulated their ideas about the construction of families and of the love, affection, and disputes that arise among family members. No other bodily substance comes close to attaining this level of significance as a marker of relationship in everyday conversations, although semen and breast milk also matter for creating relatedness. Inherited from one's father in this way of reckoning kinship, *khun* is of crucial importance in the development of a child's behavior and temperament, especially for male children. *Khun's* effects, in my experience, often come up in reference to bad behavior, partly as a way of distancing oneself from actions that inspire shame or blame. I have heard it repeated in many contexts: *"Khun ka asar hota hi hai"* ("Blood, after all, leaves its impression"). I do not claim that this statement will hold universally in North India, or even in Lucknow, because there is significant potential for variation across lines of caste and religion. My experience of these informal statements is most firmly rooted in upper-caste, middle-class Hindu and Muslim families, in which such thinking remains quite prevalent.

Higher-status families have more at stake in justifying their dominance over lower-status families through the concept of blood and for claiming exclusive rights through connections of blood. Still, other scholars have reported such sentiments as a reason for not pursuing adoption (Bhargava 2005, Bharadwaj 2003). The idea of *khun* has been explored extensively in popular culture in ways that both promote and critique the idea of *khun* as a predictor of behavior.

Khun and crime take center stage in one of the great classics of Indian cinema. Director Raj Kapoor's 1951 film *Awara* (*The Vagabond*)—starring Pritviraj Kapoor, Nargis, and Raj Kapoor—revolves around the idea of blood (*khun*) versus environment in how children turn out as they mature. Even though the film was released more than seventy years ago, it continues to circulate and to serve as an important touchpoint across multigenerational families. The film explicitly espouses the power of nurture and social structure to influence the outcome of a child's life but concludes with the hope that the vagabond in question will reform and turn out to be the respectable person he rightfully should have been based on his heritage through *khun*.

Awara opens with Judge Raghunath claiming that he has no children (*aulad*) and with a flashback to when he cast out his pregnant wife after she had been kidnapped by the *daku* (*dacoit/ robber*) Jagga. On learning that the newly abducted woman is pregnant, Jagga laughs and says that the judge accused him of being a robber because his father and grandfather were both robbers. His fault was in being the progeny (*aulad*) of robbers: "Her husband said that the progeny (*aulad*) of respectable families are always respectable and the progeny (*aulad*) of robbers are always robbers. Now I will see how Mr. Lawyer's progeny turns out."[15]

In this rendition, the children of respectable people are destined to turn out well because of their biological background, and the children of robbers are condemned to follow in the footsteps of their forefathers. Stereotypes abound regarding the nature (*svabhav* or *fitrat*) of people belonging to particular castes, in terms not only of their occupations but also their tendencies to be clever, or stupid, or greedy (Sinha and Sinha 1967; Berreman 1960). Such traits tend to be seen as inborn and impervious to change, despite one's best efforts.

In *Awara*, Judge Raghunath's wife leaves for Bombay (Mumbai), where she raises her only son, Raj, in destitution, while somehow managing to send him to school. Eventually, he is forced to leave school and falls under the influence of none other than Jagga, who initiates him into a life of crime and presents himself as a substitute father. After years of being in and out of jail, the adult Raj gets released, only to return to petty crime. As in the film *Aulad* (discussed in chapter 2), the most impassioned ideological and moral preaching in the film happens in the courtroom. Raj finally gets the opportunity there to face representatives of the law and his father, Judge Raghunath. Raj does not ask for forgiveness, nor does he deny his bad deeds. He takes the platform before the court to berate the assembly about his wayward life, saying, "I didn't get the germs of crime in my blood (*khun*) from my mother and father. I got them from the filthy gutter that flows next to our filthy little rented home. . . . Let it not be so that one day you . . . and you . . . and you . . . and your child should stand in this cage and say that the blood of a very respectable father is running in my veins. Once upon a time, I, too, like your children, was cheerful and innocent"[16] (Kapoor et al., *Awara* 2:38:00–2:40:00, 2000). In the end, Judge Raghunath acknowledges Raj as his son, and Raj receives a short jail sentence for his crimes. Despite Raj's pleas to the contrary, the lingering message of the film remains Judge Raghunath's repeated and repeatedly echoed assertion that the nature of one's character is determined by birth.

Bhargava also notes the concerns that people considering adoption have about available children's backgrounds, the nature of their "nature." She reports sayings like "The child of a thief will become a thief and nothing else" (*"Chor ka baccha to chor hi banega"*) (2005, 68). In everyday talk in Lucknow, I have often heard people compare the content of human nature with the behavior of various species of animals. People argue that just as animals have their own inbred nature to attack, or to eat meat, or to be stubborn, which varies according to their species and breed, so do human beings have certain inborn tendencies that incline them toward particular ways of behaving. Expecting animals to change from the nature they are born with is foolish at best and dangerous at worst, and so is expecting any permanent change in a human being's nature. Efforts to bring about such change are ultimately futile, and one has to learn instead either how to avoid trouble or how to deal with a person's nature (*svabhav* or *fitrat*) as it is.

The implications of such thinking for adoption seem to be quite dire. Bhargava notes that "families that register for adoption often request a child belonging to the upper caste or class . . . *'acchhi family se baccha chahiye'* ('we want a child from a good family,' where 'good family' implies upper class or caste") (2005, 67). When families articulate the desire for a child from a "good family," those words carry the weight of available children's reputations in agencies. These children have been abandoned; they must be unwanted for a reason. The most commonly cited reasons are that they were born from a nonmarital sexual liaison, that they were born female in a family that desired males, or that they were born into a family too poor to consider taking on another mouth to feed, even though abortion is legal and readily available in India. None of these reasons indicates an abandoned child's origins in a "good family." Children are much more likely to move from poor and low-caste families to much wealthier and higher-caste families through adoption within India or beyond. People often sense these social distances through locally perceptible, though sometimes mistaken, differences in features and skin color between adoptive parents and children. Adopting a child from within the extended family would negate these differences and concerns to a measurable extent but could create other conflicts about the child's loyalties. With trends toward smaller families and a higher prevalence of birth control use, there are relatively fewer children available for permanent transfer within so-called "good families."

As a form of child circulation and as one possible way of dealing with the pain associated with childlessness resulting from infertility, child adoption—particularly the adoption of strangers—has not fulfilled culturally valued markers of relatedness in North India, particularly for people of high status. Legal adoptions bring about the most obvious and egregious violations of ideals of shared substance, while other forms of adoption may make it easier for people to adopt while concealing their actions from others. Representations of adoption as a type of family formation are also changing in popular culture, as films like the hit *Baghban* (Chopra 2003, "The Gardener"), starring Amitabh Bachchan, Hema Malini, and Salman Khan, demonstrate and provide opportunities for families to discuss the implications of adoption. In *Baghban*, an elderly husband and wife who have invested all their wealth in raising their children find themselves in need of financial support in their retirement. Despite having four biological sons, they have no one willing to care for them; that is, until the unrelated child whose education they supported from childhood onward finds out and willingly takes on the responsibility of looking after them. Representations like this and the positive press for celebrities who adopt unrelated children may contribute, over time, to more openness about child adoption.

Historically, Indian law and social practice have stratified the ability of Indians wishing to adopt unrelated children to do so, depending on their religious identity and class status. Adoption certainly is an option for some couples suffering from infertility in India, but not for all. The reasons why some couples suffering from infertility may either dismiss adoption as a possibility or consider it a less desirable way of creating a family with children vary from theories of relatedness, to concerns about the implications of having adoption become public knowledge, to legal limitations. Which of these concerns or combination of concerns takes on utmost importance depends largely on a couple's position in Indian society and their confidence in their abilities to deal with the challenges they see as arising in adoptive families. Some couples clearly have the confidence to become "moral pioneers" in obtaining children through the use of ARTs, including by using donated gametes or by adopting a child. Yet many among these pioneers do so with the hope of shielding their actions from others to spare themselves and their child or children from the stigma associated with defying reproductive expectations. The practice of private adoptions carried out in collaboration with government employees and, sometimes, medical professionals, which circumvents the normal home visits and paper trail associated with legal adoption, although legally dubious, does fit into this model of becoming pioneers in secret—quietly defying social expectations.

NOTES

1. Quotes are drawn from interactions in Lucknow over the years of this study. This chapter also includes references to my fieldnotes and journal entries composed, as well as formal interactions conducted during the same time.

2. Show information and selected episodes available online at http://www.zeetv.com/shows/jhansi-ki-rani/, accessed May 24, 2021.

3. Ahmad (1975) used this phrase, which aligned with contemporary demographic approaches, such as Knowledge, Attitudes, and Practices models used to study health and fertility around the world.

4. Central Adoption Resource Authority. Ministry of Women & Child Development, Government of India, accessed April 12, 2022. http://cara.nic.in/about/about_cara.html . See also CARA, *Shared Stories*, August 5, 2015.

5. Central Adoption Resource Authority. Ministry of Women & Child Development, Government of India. http://cara.nic.in/resource /adoption_Stattistics.html, accessed May 25, 2021.

6. Central Adoption Resource Authority. Ministry of Women & Child Development, Government of India. http://cara.nic.in/about/about_cara .html accessed April 12, 2022.

7. A pseudonym.

8. National Family Health Survey, India. International Institute for Population Sciences. Key Findings from NFHS-3, accessed April 13, 2022. http://rchiips.org/nfhs/factsheet.shtml. In the 2005–2006 NFHS-3, 59.1 percent of births took place outside of institutions, with far more births at home in rural areas than in urban areas (Key Indicators Fact Sheet).

9. Central Adoption Resource Authority. Ministry of Women & Child Development, Government of India. Success Stories. accessed April 13, 2022. http://cara.nic.in/glimpse/sucess_story.html.

10. Chandrachud, D. Y. Bombay Hight Court. "In the Matter of Adoption of Payal alias Sharinee Vinay Pathak vs. Nil." http://airwebworld .com/content/viewjudgment/ViewJudgement.php?anCardId=36714&txt =juvenile%20justice%20act%20adoption, accessed August 6, 2015.

11. "Sushmita Can Keep Her Baby." *Indian Express*, January 14, 2010, http://indianexpress.com/article/cities/mumbai/sushmita-can-keep-her -baby/, accessed April 12, 2022.

12. With reference to personal laws, marriage and divorce have been the most thoroughly examined in scholarship. For more on the administration of personal laws in India, see especially Vatuk (2009) and Williams (2006).

13. *"Beta banaane se beta nahin banta, na beti, khun ka rishta."*

14. *Gazette of India*, 2015.

15. In Hindi: *"Is ke pati ne kaha tha ki sharifon ki aulad hamesha sharif hoti hain aur chor daku ki aulad hamesha chor daku hoti hain. Ab main dekhunga vakil saahab ki aulad kaisi hoti hai."*

16. "Germs": Literally insects or worms (*keeṛe*), also used to refer to cavities, some other disease-causing agents, and sperm.

—ɯᴗ—

CONCLUSION

Reproductive Openings and Reproductive Justice in
Contemporary India

IN THE EARLY PART OF my fieldwork in Lucknow, I understood the term *aulad* as simply a synonym for the word *baccha,*
which in everyday usage covers the meanings conveyed by the
English words "fetus," "infant," and "child." Women in Lucknow's
Gehumandi settlement showed me the richness of the concept of
aulad as an ideal of children who shared bodily substances understood through idioms of blood and, to some extent, biology, and
as a major key to family continuity. They helped me understand
the depth of fights for gender equality and equity in language and
culture by questioning whether or not *aulad* must be male, even
though the term is grammatically female and plural. They made
clear the stakes of understandings of *aulad* for the lives of women
as women, mothers, and members of their marital households, as
well as the transformative potential of working for other visions
of kinship through the everyday work of becoming family. Representations of *aulad, khun* (blood), and the *sasural* (in-laws' place)
in films, songs, and other popular culture and their echoes in
women's accounts of society and of their personal experiences af-
firmed the deep resonances of these intertwined concepts across
generations as well as the long-term struggles that hover close to
them. I came to see the production of *aulad* not only as a physical

process of creating progeny but also as a tournament of meanings to be created, contested, and reproduced along with children. Women suffering because of infertility sometimes mentioned the importance of having sons, but they tended to focus more on the centrality of being able to have a child of one's "own" (*apna*). That is, they worked toward getting a child that either had an appropriate, accepted biological connection to the family or that could be presented as such within the larger family and community.

In the context of North India, the problem of infertility poses unique opportunities for women and their confidantes to reflect on the importance of *aulad*. For women suffering because of their unfulfilled desire for children, the concept of *aulad* shapes their approaches to dealing with infertility. It also influences the likelihood that particular information about their reproductive quests will be revealed to or concealed from other family members, friends, and neighbors. I heard common ideals about producing *aulad* from women across religious, economic, and caste boundaries. Regardless of religious identification, women in Lucknow expressed similar ideological commitments about the significance of *aulad* for families. They demonstrated similar understandings of *aulad* and similar contestations of the concept amid changing gender relations and economic conditions. Yet, their abilities to pursue and fulfill their reproductive desires varied, as I found by talking with women, medical professionals, and social workers, especially at infertility clinics, charity health camps, and adoption centers.

While people asserted the common desperation of women suffering from infertility, in Lucknow, class and religious background structured the options available to people searching for children to join their families. Religious doctrine and practice influenced perceptions of specific ritual reasons for having children and the possible ways of obtaining children that people can claim as their own (*apna*). Yet, religious doctrine and practice do not completely explain the differences that I have described, primarily between Hindus and Muslims. Muslims I interviewed did not express less desire for children, or for *aulad* in particular, than did non-Muslims. The legacies of the colonial structure of family law divided by religious identification and the invisibility of minority infertility have had the effect of limiting options for adoption and other reproductive strategies to alleviate infertility for Indians belonging to minority religious groups and people living in poverty. Especially in the case of Muslims, financial factors and perceptions of social discrimination create additional constraints on their options for obtaining children they could call their own.

Women I met in Lucknow by and large did not seem to focus on contributing numbers to the nation, or warriors to a battle, as some strains of national discourse about population suggest, particularly in the case of Muslims. However, they were encouraged to think about contributing members to the family line (*vansh/khandaan*). The realities of everyday life placed them in close contact with members of the extended family, whether or not they were residing together. Awareness of neighborhood talk—whether framed as conversation (*baat, baatchit,* or *guftugu*) or gossip (*gapshap*)—also mattered. Local attitudes contribute much greater immediacy and account for much more motivation in the pursuit of children than do the speeches and slogans of politicians and religious leaders. Conversations with people who had not personally dealt with infertility helped me situate the local dynamics of the social context in which women experience infertility. This is not to say that demographic competition does not exist, but, in the case of women in Lucknow, local concerns, not national ones, were primary drivers in the quests of people seeking to remedy reproductive absences. And, when broken down by religion, the most recent national data show that overall fertility rates among Muslims are falling more quickly than among people in other religious categories (Padmanabhan 2015; Singh 2020).

As I look back on the ways that women in Lucknow hid reproduction during the time of my fieldwork, I am reminded of
how some of these practices continue in daily life and extend far
beyond concealing infertility problems from others. Many Indian women take small and elaborate steps to hide the existence
of sexual activity as insinuated by dating before marriage, by
birth-control devices or medications, and by concrete evidence
of sexual activity. They may also keep pregnancy hidden for as
long as possible under a loose tunic or behind the folds of a sari.
Public displays of affection still garner criticism. And yet, these
are not the only currents of sexual expression or of reproduction
in contemporary India. In urban areas, where over 30 percent
of Indians live, and especially in large cities such as New Delhi
and Mumbai, some young people are testing and pushing the
boundaries of openness to wear revealing clothing, to date and
kiss in public, to have live-in relationships before marriage, and to
choose their own marital partners (Mody 2008). Such actions do
not go on without criticism from relatives, or from self-appointed
moral police, and may involve a host of negative consequences,
especially for women.

People can and do cite verified cases and rumors about rapes;
murders; ostracism from home, family, and jobs; and other less
severe yet important negative consequences incurred by those
who have refused to comply with gendered expectations about
women's dress, conduct, sexual expression, partnering, and reproduction (Chowdhry 2007). Still, some women and others refuse to capitulate to conventions reinforced by these stories that
continue to occur and to circulate. The liberalization of the Indian economy since the 1990s has created new possibilities for the
consumption of commodities and ideas from all over the world.
Expanding employment and speed of communication have created room for some young people to experiment in ways their
parents might never have expected. Economic liberalization and
technological innovations have also led to new possibilities for

Indian bodies to be drawn into transnational reproductive mar-
kets, not only through adoption but also through applications of
assisted reproductive technologies (ARTs) for gamete donation
and surrogacy.

The idea of hiding reproduction immediately draws attention
to issues of visibility in reproduction and may evoke images of
pregnant bellies bared to a photographer's lens, or of photographs
or videos of fetal sonograms. Such images have become ubiquitous in mass-media representations of reproduction and in self-
presentations on social media as people share their reproductive
journeys online. I have focused on practices that hide the specif-
ics of reproduction in the interest of alleviating infertility because
of its stigmatizing effects. My presentation of struggles to make
families in Lucknow may inspire comparison with other contexts
of family-making in places with related demographic profiles,
concerns, and trajectories, such as China. Their similar yet distinct histories of family structures, patriarchy, and son preference
promise productive intersections, but cultural and political differences also necessitate care in comparison. Other readers may
find a comparison with other contexts with South Asian diaspora
communities interesting or may be inspired to reflect on contexts
they find most familiar.

Connecting the dots to examine how pathways of local and
global inequality and power influence the particulars of what I
have described in Lucknow provides crucially important context
for situating reproductive experiences. Reproductive flows across
India and from India to other countries have significant implications for understanding the field within which reproduction
happens, and these flows will impact the ways people in India
understand concealing and revealing reproduction in the future.
Media certainly has a role to play in ideological change, but I
am talking more about the stuff of making the future through
the bioavailability (Cohen 2005) of Indian human resources
to globally wealthy reproductive exiles (Inhorn and Shrivastav

2010). The materiality of bodies, bodily substances, and economic resources engaged in making families in India, not only for people in India but also for people around the world, points to ethical quandaries that may inspire critical reflection on what will be at stake in desires to create kinship among people seeking family now and in future generations. New technologies, such as ARTs, can challenge the existing social order but can also be used as new tools to reinforce old ideals. World Population Day still garners national attention every July, with campaigns marking the day and prominent members of society making public statements, now including on social media, about the perceived need to curb reproduction and control population. The ideas of India as a crowded country and population as a problem continue to reverberate strongly, even as fertility rates fall.

EXPECTING IN LUCKNOW: ASPIRATIONS FOR WOMEN'S LIVES

Recent data on sex ratios in India demonstrate the continuing—and, in some cases, widening—gaps between the life chances of male and female children. There are fewer "missing girls" (Sen 1990, 2013) in some regions than others, but the general pattern holds across India. In Uttar Pradesh, the Sample Registration System Statistical Report of 2018 tallies only 880 girls per 1,000 boys at birth, lower than the national average of 899 girls per 1,000 boys.[1] Despite the existence of vibrant, diverse, and long-standing feminist movements in India, security of life with a female body can come under threat at all stages of life. While girls and women are making great strides in educational and economic achievement, the tentative nature of women's security relative to that of men continues across the life course for all but the most privileged. There are many critical junctures at which women can come to be seen by others as disposable, no longer worthy of life, whether because of their female bodies or because they attempt to make their own life decisions. Many of these moments revolve around sexual activity, marriage, and reproduction. Regardless of their religious identification, the most basic expectations for the vast majority of women in North India include getting married, usually to a man chosen by other family members, becoming mothers, and taking the primary responsibility for raising their child(ren). The possibility of opting out of or remaking these expectations is more daunting for women than for men, even though there are no guarantees that women wish to follow this prescribed life course, nor that they will be successful in reproduction if they do.

For most women, their local social environment through family members in their natal and marital households, the consciousness of neighbors and "society," and representations of mothers and children in popular culture fundamentally shape their reproductive desires. In my early days in Lucknow in 2000–2001, I asked young, unmarried people whether they wanted to have children. I remember being met with blank stares and silence. Once they broke through the shock, they would almost invariably answer with some form of "Why not?" or "What kind of question is that?" Choosing not to have children was clearly not an option that most had ever considered. Over the years I have spent in Lucknow, I have begun to hear more dissenting voices—a few women here and there who refuse to marry and may or may not seek to adopt a child without a spouse, men who tell their wives that children will cramp their lifestyle, and women who reject childbearing in favor of social work. Such sentiments may create more social space for infertile couples, but much depends on the very intimate contexts of homes and neighborhoods in which families are built, with or without children.

Among both Hindus and Muslims, infertility often provided an opportunity for women and their husbands to renegotiate intimacies within their marital households, bringing spouses closer together in their common endeavor to obtain children.

Women I interviewed in clinics appeared to be the most successful—they had achieved cooperation and financial resources
from their husbands and often in-laws or other family members
to visit the clinic in search of a solution to their fertility problems.
Stories such as the one in the *Times of India* about Rasoolan, the
daughter-in-law allegedly set on fire for her failure to conceive,
and stories from women about friends, relatives, and neighbors
suggest that household strife and harassment of women can result
from infertility. The stories women shared in infertility clinics
show that the unremitting torture of infertile and/or childless
women in everyday life need not be as universal as some media
representations suggest. Still, the potential for disaster cannot
be dismissed, and the circulation of such accounts adds to fear
of infertility, which can influence marital patterns and fertility
desires and intentions, as well as add urgency to seeking infertility treatment.

While I have included dissenting opinions about the centrality of becoming a mother to women's lives in India, these mostly
represent the voices of elite women whose privilege creates distance from the realities of most women's lives in extended families with strong expectations and reproductive aspirations. I am
still haunted by this statement from a woman I interviewed in
an infertility clinic, whose sentiments were echoed by women
in Lucknow time and again: "Whatever happens, to become a
mother is the most important job (*kaam*). . . . The one who has
nobody. . . . That poor lady, outsiders say. The one who doesn't
have any [children] learns what their importance (*ahamiyat*)
is."[2] The pressures on women not only to become mothers but to
produce desired children for their extended families are significant. People across various social locations meet the precarities
that emerge in their reproductive journeys, whether due to hormonal problems, azoospermia, low wages, or familial strife, with
persistence and creativity. Women in Lucknow have taught me
that even when confronted with reproductive challenges, many

people will muster their own emotional and social resources in their search for children, remaking intimacies within their marriages and extended families in the process.

REPRODUCTIVE EXILES AND UNDESIRABLE INDIANS

India became a major destination for medical tourism in the early twenty-first century, including for infertility treatment and surrogacy (Haimowitz and Sinha 2010). The practice of surrogacy spread and garnered attention from prospective users, journalists, ethicists, and entrepreneurs after my main fieldwork period. The number of clinics offering surrogacy and the international renown of such clinics expanded exponentially, eventually leading India to address the implications of becoming a receiving country for reproductive tourists, otherwise known as reproductive exiles (Inhorn 2015; Inhorn and Shrivastav 2010), from around the world by taking steps to restrict or end crossborder reproduction.[3] Global and local inequalities and the proliferation of ARTs complicate the legal, ethical, and cultural implications of the creation and transfer of children and of other biological materials used in assisted reproduction, such as used embryos (Bharadwaj 2008), in contemporary India, whether the scope is international or domestic. Scholars have focused on representations of the women who have given birth through commercial surrogacy and have interviewed many of them as well as medical staff, clients, and others at length (Deomampo 2013, 2016; Majumdar 2013, 2018; Pande 2009a, 2009b, 2010, 2014; Rudrappa 2015; Saravanan 2018; Vora 2009a, 2009b, 2015). However, the roles that local understandings of kinship and internal social discrimination play in who becomes a surrogate—in terms of religious, caste, and regional background, not just economic class—have so far only been partially documented (Sama Resource Group for Women and Health 2010, 2012). Although it is impossible to know precisely how many children have been born through surrogacy in India, transnational movement makes some accounting possible. Estimates suggest that they numbered in the range of hundreds to up to two thousand per year (Bhatia 2012; DasGupta and Das Dasgupta 2014).

The impact of ARTs on reproductive desires and practices in India continues to be a topic of emergent importance, particularly in the context of shifting practices of surrogacy and adoption (DasGupta and Das Dasgupta 2014; Howell 2006; Mohanty, Ahn, and Chokkanathan 2014; Unisa, Pujari, and Ganguly 2012). Surrogacy and adoption have, so far, mostly received scholarly attention at the level of transnational transfers. With the suspension of transnational commercial surrogacy in 2015 and continuing legislative moves on bans and/or regulation, the ultimate long-term future of crossborder commercial surrogacy in India seems dubious.[4] Surrogacy practice and the use of other ARTs continue domestically, and clinics with equipment, staff, and networks are finding other ways to participate in transnational reproduction (Pande 2021; Rudrappa 2017). Many stories remain to be discovered and told—by those bold enough not to hide them or at least bold enough to tell them behind veils of confidentiality and pseudonyms—by people who have created families domestically in India using these methods.

The media and scholarly attention garnered by transnational surrogacy far outstrips its numerical prevalence, especially when compared to the millions of infertile people living in India who could not even begin to consider surrogacy as a way of making families for financial, cultural, and other reasons. Still, the debates around surrogacy have created opportunities to reflect on infertility treatment in India in general and on other reproductive practices. In a larger sense, ARTs and specific applications of them, such as surrogacy, provide an opening to reconsider how and why people make kin and perhaps to imagine new ways of doing kinship (Singh 2014, 2018). In Lucknow, women's perspectives on infertility contribute to illuminating the rich cultural contexts within which children are created and/or transferred to foreigners; Indians settled abroad; and Indians living in India through surrogacy, adoption, or other forms of child circulation. They also have broader comparative importance for evaluating the ethical implications of reproductive technologies and point to ways in which reproductive technologies and legal regulation can amplify existing injustices embedded in institutions and through the ways people in the contemporary world value human lives in particular local and national contexts. The movement of bodies and bodily substances, including reproductive substances, through transnational surrogacy has added a new dimension to scholarly analyses of how the contours of reproductive labor contribute to global stratified reproduction.

TECHNOLOGY, SECRECY, AND MODERNITY

The North Indian cultural concept of *aulad* has varied and contested meanings that help women in Lucknow imagine how successful reproduction looks and feels. The problem of infertility and the availability of several different methods for resolving involuntary childlessness present unique challenges and opportunities for those suffering from infertility. People dealing with infertility must confront and work around questions about how kin relations and attachment are generated among children, parents, and extended families, through locally salient categories such as "blood," caste, religion, genetics, and care. The availability of a wide range of methods—medical, spiritual, and kinship-based—for dealing with infertility and childlessness presents them with the opportunity to become "moral pioneers" (following Rapp 1988, 1999). They may create novel forms of relatedness, approximating old ideals of relatedness by concealing their use of strategies such as biomedical infertility treatment and/or infant adoption, or settling into a life without their "own" children. For women suffering because of their unfulfilled desire for children, the concept of *aulad* shapes their approaches to dealing with in-fertility and the likelihood that they will disclose particular infor-mation about their reproductive quests to other family members, friends, and neighbors.

ARTs, including in vitro fertilization, join lower-tech strat-egies such as donor insemination in the expanding landscape of biomedical infertility treatment. Lower-tech options such as donor insemination can be transformed by their location in the infertility clinic from a threat to paternity, family unity, and the social order into a potentially acceptable way to save marriages and families under the veil of secrecy. Even the topic of donor in-semination has lost enough stigma to garner a Bollywood film—a comedy—called *Vicky Donor* (Lulla et al. 2012). Control over the method of procurement and the flow of information (and se-men) in clinics aid this transformation. The biomedical infertility clinic offers options for procreative creativity that can be hidden from others with relative ease. It enables people suffering from infertility to avoid potential social stigma by approximating their ideals of the production of *aulad* and projecting an ideal image to others in their social world, regardless of the details of how their babies were made.

Disparities in access to fertility-enhancing technologies, the realities of urban living, and the surveillance of neighbors and family members mean that not all women are equally able to achieve secrecy in their reproductive pursuits. The burqa and other means of veiling the female body have the potential to aid Muslim women, in particular, in this endeavor in all but their most local contexts, in which details of their movement, shoes, jewelry, the style of the burqa or veil, and specific movements would likely undo their anonymity. Yet these concealing forms of dress can also become an object of scorn in clinics, signifying Muslim women as antimodern "others" and as bad patients.

There were women in Lucknow who contributed their per-spectives and experiences to this project to voice doubts about the importance of children to a successful life, but they were few and far between. Women who were willing to openly pursue and acknowledge children procured through adoption or through the use of ARTs were also few. Much more common were women willing to be moral pioneers in private but to project an image of a conventional family to others, often including other family members and "society" in general. By and large, ARTs helped women to display their adherence to established reproductive norms— in some cases, while violating them—rather than to openly defy them. In this sense, undertaking adoption would require a level of boldness in facing family and "society" that women who used ARTs to fulfill their own and their marital families' desires for children hoped to avoid.

Bharadwaj (2003, 1867) has argued that in India, adoption is not a viable option because it puts infertility on display, while the use of ARTs in clinics can be hidden through silence. While this may hold true when silence can be achieved, Bharadwaj shows that even for well-to-do couples receiving treatments in private clinics in the late 1990s, achieving silence about infertility treatment required many complex maneuvers and the cooperation of medical staff. Some couples are better equipped for success in achieving secrecy than others. Two decades later, the ubiquity of cell phones and their increasing sophistication is creating new potential for secrecy in communication and in gathering fertility-related information, but it also creates new possibilities for discovery through the digital trail of text messages and browser histories. Still, some disclosure may be necessary for recruiting the practical help needed to facilitate trips to a clinic and/or to manage the questions of curious neighbors, family, and friends.

With the proliferation of smartphones, more affordable internet access, and social media in South Asia, new opportunities have been created for women to learn, to find resources, and to network with others. The expansion of these technologies has contributed to fostering a #MeToo movement in India (Philipose and Kesavan 2019) and to sharing reproductive health information, such as basic educational materials on menstruation, online.[5] As in most of the world, access to technology also comes with perceived peril from people who would limit young people's access to information and to potential romantic partners. Continuing to document the effects of technology on the lives of women of reproductive age and of children whose status as acceptable family members—worthy of being called one's "own"—could be called into question will remain an important task for understanding how and why families are being made in India.

What has not been possible in kinship for many generations is becoming more possible through technology, but only for those people who have the financial and emotional resources to do so. Even then, secrecy may be threatened by modern legal institutions in which paternity can be defined through DNA and tests can be performed to confirm or deny genetic links in disputes. The availability of ARTs continues to increase in both the private and government sectors in India. ARTs provide a new way of achieving an old goal in relation to infertility—finding ways to present one's community with *aulad* without creating doubt about that child's origin. The internet and social media can offer much in terms of finding resources, but that depends on online materials being up to date, which is not guaranteed. And it is not always strictly necessary. When I revisited one of the government infertility clinics where I had conducted research in 2015, I found that the waiting room of the new unit into which the clinic had settled featured a prominent poster board. Attached was a list of local adoption resources with phone numbers that would be visible to anyone in the clinic. It was a small gesture, but that list provided a potential escape from the travails of infertility treatment, an indicator of possible paths patients could discuss with others in the clinic or could follow out of the clinic, and perhaps a justification for another way of making a family.

AULAD AND REPRODUCTIVE FUTURES

The vast majority of social-science research on reproductive desires in India has focused on high fertility, rather than on infertility, and has explicated the significance of region, caste, religion,
economics, and education on fertility levels. Religion, in particular, has become a central focus of political debate about reproduction in contemporary India, but without reference to the
realities of health disparities and social discrimination in everyday life and too often leaving out the deeply intimate emotional
core of reproduction. Centering women's reproductive desires
and bringing together perspectives of fertility and infertility experiences, as they intersect with the social and cultural factors
that influence how people go about finding children for families,
demonstrates some of the complexities of reproduction in this
context.

    People suffering from infertility in Lucknow attempted to
fulfill their desires for children through strategies ranging from
biomedical treatments, including ARTs, to adoption and other
forms of child circulation. Religion, class, and consciousness of
social stigma shape the experiences of people suffering from infertility who seek novel ways to actualize or approximate their
goal of acquiring *aulad* and how they encounter and cocreate
aulad as a cultural category along the way. This category provides crucial context to understand the importance of fertility
and the threat of infertility in Lucknow. The meanings and uses
of *aulad* illustrate how ideologies and practices of family, kinship,
and the future influence reproductive desires and practices more
broadly in India. Thinking with *aulad* and its contestations could
help in formulating comparative questions for other places where
the proliferation of technologies to control, enhance, and limit
fertility ignites debates about gender, kinship, and belonging in
families, as well as in larger cultural, demographic, and national
categories. While emphasizing the nuances of reproduction in

Lucknow, it also points to the benefits of bringing together demographic and ethnographic perspectives to illuminate the relationships between fertility and infertility that are emblematic of the fertility-infertility dialectic (Inhorn 1994, 23) and that so profoundly impact lived experiences of reproduction in North India and around the world (Johnson et al. 2018, 649).

Activist groups in the United States have been advocating for going beyond the often individual focus of programs on reproductive health and rights to examine collective issues through bringing together the frames of human rights and social justice, far beyond the dominant US focus on abortion (ACRJ 2005; Ross 2006; Ross and Solinger 2017; Ross et al. 2017; Davis 2019; Luna and Luker 2013; Luna 2020; Scott 2021). Since the late 1990s, the movement for reproductive justice in the United States has pushed advocacy on reproduction beyond abortion politics and individuals to larger collectivities to address reproductive oppressions that stand in the way of achieving reproductive justice. As awareness of the movement's contributions to theory, practice, and advocacy has grown, so has scholars' engagement with it on a wide range of reproductive topics, including infertility, mainly grounded in and focused on the experiences of people of color in the United States, and especially of Black women (Barnes and Fledderjohann 2020; Ceballo 2017; Ceballo, Graham, and Hart 2015; Inhorn, Ceballo, and Nachtigall 2009; Luna 2018).

While specific to the United States, the reproductive justice movement and its core ideas provide a productive model for asking good questions and thinking about what the units of analysis ought to be to describe the contexts within which people in other places could seek locally meaningful reproductive justice. The capaciousness of the framework and its emphasis on addressing the root causes of reproductive injustices (Davis 2019) give it ample scope to serve as one approach to recognizing, understanding, and working to transform similar situations elsewhere in the world. What might reproductive justice look like for people living in India? This scholarly conversation has only just begun (Bailey 2011; Chandra, Satish, and Center for Reproductive Rights, 2019; Heitmeyer and Unnithan 2015; Nandagiri 2019; Saravanan 2018; Unnithan and Pigg 2014; Singh 2020), and it is bound to be a long one, with conflicting priorities that will not be resolved easily in a country with deep inequalities, internal and external pressures to focus on the numerical size and shape of future generations, and prejudices that can easily make their way into reproductive policy, healthcare systems, and clinical encounters.

The continuing sex ratio differences in India are often discussed through reference to "missing girls" (Sen 1990), "female feticide," or "son preference," all phrases commonly used and critiqued in demographic, gender studies, and other academic literature. The states with the most "missing girls" are among the most prosperous in India, where technologies to determine sex before birth are readily available and financially within reach for many people (Patel 2007b). Specific ideas about the sex of *aulad* and patterns of kinship, marriage, and inheritance continue to contribute to making female children less desired, even among childless people. These shared understandings manifest in practices such as sex-selective abortion, infanticide, abandonment, and bias against girls in the distribution of food and medical care. While ideologies and practices both shift and persist, this issue merits continued consideration as the Indian economy expands, the cost of living increases, and people continue to come to grips with the effects of pandemic disease and climate change.

Although I argue that ideologies about *aulad* are shared across religious lines, Islam specifically teaches against practices intended to eliminate girl children. Muslim women in Lucknow rarely cited this teaching to me, unless it was specifically part of an educational program. Practices to eliminate female children—actual or potential—have been suggested to be less prevalent, although not absent, among Indian Muslims, as compared to among members of other religious communities (Khan 2010).

As changing marriage practices among Indian Muslims increase the pressure on the parents of daughters to spend large amounts of money for wedding ceremonies and gifts, these patterns may well trend toward greater discrimination against girls. In ideological terms, as Muslim women activists in Lucknow argued, Islamic teachings present some scope to argue for the value of children across sex differences and to raise the prospects for girls and women through small, everyday decisions about education, health, marriage, and reproduction. Yet, for people from backgrounds marking them as reproductive "others" because of their religious, caste, or class identities, reproduction happens within a larger context that devalues the lives they struggle to create and sustain. Creating the most valued family forms is most achievable from the most privileged social positions. Ramberg (2014) documents an alternative strategy in South India for making women structural sons by dedicating daughters to a goddess through *devadasi*, a practice apparently nearing its end by means of social and legal reforms that narrow acceptable kinship. At the same time, historical scholarship on South Asia provides evidence of other ways families have been made in India that could gain renewed legitimacy.

The invisible infertile in India are invisible not only because infertility is not a priority for a national and international reproductive health apparatus still focused on reducing birth rates, and not only because infertility data is difficult to tease out of large-scale demographic studies. Many infertile people would rather evade recognition of their creativity in kinship, presenting challenges for rectifying silences in the data. Still, finding safe ways to share stories can be a powerful tool for normalizing infertility experiences. Women I met in infertility clinics frequently told me that they had thought they were alone in their infertility struggles until they made their way to the clinic and found themselves surrounded by other women hoping to become mothers.

Reproductive disruption includes, at its heart, an impetus to action but without a single specific direction. The idea of disruption implies ideals and desires, which could inspire attempts to preserve or approximate those ideals and desires using available resources. In Lucknow, most women I encountered in infertility clinics were working toward finding ways to meet patriarchal family visions of appropriate reproduction that made sense within their ideas about the way kinship ought to work. However, as their efforts failed to produce results, they also reconsidered these ideals and thought about ways to get around them. If few women I met had reached a point of rejecting motherhood or biological relationship, it may be that those ideologies were too strong to dismiss. Or perhaps I had reached them too early in their journeys.

Some women had begun, though, to think about the opportunities for creativity, innovation, and defiance of social norms— open or covert—that reproductive disruption in the forms of infertility, the loss of children, and/or the absence of sons created for them. Interruptions in conventionally expected and accepted reproductive paths embody a revolutionary potential for making families that reaches far beyond infertility clinics and adoption agencies into the most intimate spaces for creating and sustaining connections among human beings within and across generations. Moral pioneers, many of them compelled by their medical, financial, and other circumstances may indeed be engaged in work that will point to new ways of imagining and creating links among human beings. That so many of them labor in secret shows how contested—and how significant—this endeavor may be for human futures.

NOTES

1. Office of the Registrar General & Census Commissioner, India. Sample Registration System Statistical Report 2018. https://censusindia

.gov.in/vital_statistics/SRS_Reports_2018.html, chap. 3, p. 56, accessed May 27, 2021.

2. Quote from a Sikh woman undergoing infertility treatment, group conversation, Lucknow infertility clinic, 2007.

3. See, for example, Sinha (2016): "Women Have Right to Be Mothers, Not Surrogates," (Venkatesan 2016; Rabinowitz 2016).

4. See, for example, Pande (2021), Sinha (2016), Venkatesan (2016), and Rabinowitz (2016).

5. For example, a comic book is available here in multiple South Asian languages: Menstrupedia Technologies Private Limited. *Menstrupedia.* https://www.menstrupedia.com/, accessed June 9, 2021. Menstrupedia includes a blog and other information free online as well as a printed book. Gupta, Aditi, and Tuhin Paul. *Menstrupedia Comic: The Friendly Guide to Periods for Girls.* India: Menstrupedia, 2014. See also Kamini Prakash, guest editor, *Indian Journal of Gender Studies* 26, nos. 1/2 (2019), Special Issue: Narratives of Bodily Functions.

—◊—

AFTERWORD
Family Plans, Or, Waiting for Aulad

MY OBSERVATIONS ON THE RELATIONSHIPS between marriage and the birth of children come from years of conversations
with young women in India, mostly in Lucknow, but they are
also grounded in my own experience of nearly two decades (and
counting) as a daughter-in-law of a family from Uttar Pradesh
that has been settled in Lucknow since the 1970s. I hold no delusions that my own experience neatly mirrors that of some ideal
Lakhnavi woman (a woman of Lucknow)—a category that, in
the first place, cannot exist in the singular. The family into which
I married, through a "love match," rather than an arranged one,
calls itself middle class—although I see that as a nebulous classification. They base that classification mostly on my now-retired
father-in-law's career as a midlevel state government servant. The
family is Hindu and belongs to the Kshatriya (warrior) caste.
My partner, Deepak, is five years older than me. According to
traditions of his caste and social group, which he has spent most
of his life disregarding, the timing of the marriage was appropriate in terms of our ages. I had just completed the first semester
of my master's degree and was young for marriage according to
mainstream American standards, but not according to my working-class, rural origins—I was one of the first among my college

friends to get married, but one of the last among my high school friends.

In our case, to be accepted socially in Lucknow and in Deepak's family, and to spend time in the United States, required marriage. Immigration from India to the United States without marriage remains difficult and lengthy unless a person is part of a high-demand profession or can obtain a visa with a path to permanent residency through the sponsorship of a family member already settled in the United States. Deepak's family accepted me from the start and went out of their way to help me feel like part of the family. I was inquisitive, but I also acquiesced to much of their guidance about how to act with relatives, friends, and acquaintances. I did not live with them full-time, since I returned to the United States about four weeks after the marriage, which took place during the break between fall and spring semesters. Deepak followed me to Charlottesville after nine months, when I concluded a summer study trip to Lucknow.

Relatively few daughters-in-law in Lucknow encounter as much flexibility regarding their adjustment in their *sasural* (in-laws' home) as I did. My status as a foreign woman who could speak Hindi and who preferred to wear *shalwar kameez* (a tunic and loose pants, usually worn with a scarf) or the occasional sari, rather than jeans or skirts, also helped me establish myself as a legitimate part of the family. The adjustment would likely have been much more difficult had I not looked white, had I been Muslim, or had I been a Hindu of a different—especially a lower—caste. It also helped that I was the first *bahu* to enter this household, since my partner is the eldest of three children. His sister was already married, and his brother was still in university studying, so there were no other *bahus* with whom to compete for status or favors, or with whose behavior to make comparisons. There have been obvious differences between myself and most *bahus* in my in-laws' social circle—including my career path as an anthropologist employed outside of the home. Still, over

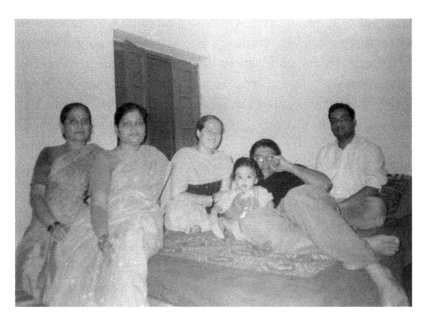

Figure 7.1. A small part of a sprawling extended family, 2003.

the years, some people within my extended Indian family and friends have come to portray me as an ideal of a *bahu*, especially in contrast to Indian women who reject or fail to live up to their in-laws' expectations. I have yet to come to grips with this, and I have many feminist dilemmas over this sort of portrayal, in which I have been deployed as an example to criticize the behavior of other women, despite the benefits that I have derived from spending at least part of my time living within a joint family.

Residence in a joint family has its ups and downs, its costs and benefits, as does any way of organizing the division of household labor. But what is most relevant to the discussion here is my experience of becoming part of a family in which the birth of children soon after marriage tends to be taken as the ordinary course of life. Deepak and I had decided that we would not even consider the possibility of children for several years after marriage because of our ambitions to pursue our careers and to travel, and because of the limitations on time and finances imposed by my pursuit of a PhD. Our own decisions were shaped to a large extent by our extreme rationality about the organization of insurance coverage, parental leave, and childcare in the United States.

My partner is by nature a very funny person, and if anyone made insinuations about our intentions or "efforts" to produce good news (*khush khabri*) implying impending childbirth, he would find some laughable way of fending off their questions. At the start of our marriage, few people inquired, and Deepak's mother was also prompt in responding to people that Holly was still studying, so let her finish her studies! As time went by, people not only started to ask more frequently about when we would have children; even my mother-in-law started to ask when I would be done with graduate school—a very bad question to ask most American doctoral students. Deepak's answers to people's queries became more and more embarrassing for the unwitting souls who dared to ask, such as "We're trying!" and "We won't have any. We've passed our expiration date!" By 2006, when we arrived in Lucknow for my long-term fieldwork, people were apparently really starting to wonder and to be somewhat concerned about my age, although I was still under thirty. Needless to say, the fact that I was doing field research on infertility did not help matters. Women being treated in infertility clinics often followed my questions about their quests for children with their own queries about my marital and fertility status. Between the questions from women with whom I interacted in fieldwork and those from Deepak's extended family and their friends, I started to become haunted by the doubt that if and when we did consider the possibility of trying to conceive, we would suffer from some sort of infertility problem.

At some point, Deepak's mother also began telling us that she didn't need new saris or money or anything else but a "gift"— by which she meant a baby, although she did not push her will through measures such as preventing the use of birth control. She would mention wanting a beautiful, fair girl similar to the daughter of an American friend of ours who was then working on a research project in Lucknow, but otherwise did not place heavy emphasis on the sex of the child, especially since Deepak kept telling her that we would not have any child at all. Other family members made occasional comments as well. One particularly outspoken uncle had a new euphemism for the process of conception every time he visited, which always included pointed references, such as "shooting the arrow," "making the goal," or "shooting the bullet." He also waxed philosophical about the meanings of children, explaining that "children are like toys for their grandparents," and that whatever sorrows my parents-in-law might have, a child would chase them away. At some point, Deepak suggested adopting a child to avoid the strains of pregnancy and dangers associated with childbirth. Nearly everyone he told in India rejected this idea. Deepak is generally very squeamish about blood and pain, and he feared that I could die while giving birth, although he did not voice this concern to his family and friends in India. I felt as if many people looked at the prospect of our children as a lab experiment, in which they were curious about what sort of compound or precipitate would develop from combining our strange and exotic elements.

As a *bahu* in my *sasural*, I measured my reactions to any difficulties with the thought that these were temporary issues, of no major consequence, and that anyway they were likely to be of short duration, since we would return to the United States at some point. My home with Deepak's family did not even remotely feel like a *sasural* in the sense of the dreaded place for daughters-in-law until Deepak's younger brother (my *devar*) got married in 2007, and then it was the behavior of his wife (my *devrani*, to whom I am *bhabhi* or *jethani*) that drove conflicts. Her constant comparisons of the way Deepak's parents treated me versus her—in terms of the expectations they had of her versus of me for helping with the household chores and attending to guests—seemed to be fueled by a presumption of the oppression of daughters-in-law in the *sasural* and her determination not to be treated unequally. Her image of the *sasural* struck me as completely incommensurate with my experience of my *sasural*. In those early days, she also never seemed to notice that I was still in school, working on my PhD, while she had completed her studies, or that I was doing research through a grant, while she worked in the home, watched television, and slept. She criticized what I wore, where I went, and so on much more than my in-laws had ever done in five years of marriage, and her comparisons took a toll on everyone. Her adjustment in the household was much more difficult than mine, perhaps because everyone expected similarity in her case, and they had expected difference in mine.

Ours was certainly an unconventional situation, since I was a strange *bahu*, but also because the younger *bahu* had a different outlook and she defied the deference and respectful behavior generally expected from *bahus* toward their parents-in-law and toward their spouse's elder brother and wife (*jeth* and *jethani*). She was the eldest in a family of three daughters, and she jumped at any chance to talk about matters of female biology, birth control, and pregnancy. She was less than subtle in her hints that she and Deepak's brother were "ready to become Uncle and Aunt" (*chacha* and *chachi*).

The waiting game never turned into household bickering, threats, or accusations of the sort that Indian women suffering from infertility sometimes narrated to me, but it may be that the way we framed our nonproduction of progeny even years after marriage encouraged family members to focus their energies on trying to convince us of the need to have a child, rather than to deride or belittle us. No one dared to ask whether there might be any physical, spiritual, or other problem, and we did not allow such questions to arise. We took the matter of children lightly but also realized that most of the people around us did not. In thinking through the reasons why friends, family members, and strangers questioned our intentions so closely and argued for the necessity of producing children, Khare's work referring to the significance of relationships among husband/wife/child comes to mind. He argues, "The parents begin to see themselves and their relationships through the child; they are to each other mainly or only that which a child's presence, now or in future, would make them to be" (1982, 166). In this understanding of the child, it is the child that ultimately creates, or re-creates, the relationship between partners. The child binds husband and wife and creates a bond of "blood" (*rakta* or *khun*) between husband and wife, without regard to other cominglings of bodily substance, food, water, and so on. The child also transforms their social identities. This sort of transformation conspicuously leaves out those without children or who make families in other ways and discounts the possibility that husband/wife relationships might be complete without the addition of a child.

Khare's analysis here can be extended further to understand the role that a child plays in families beyond marital partners. When wife becomes transformed into mother, she can also be addressed as the mother of so-and-so by others in the family, making her status less exclusive. In other words, while she is only a wife to her husband, she is the mother of so-and-so to everyone. In the rural communities where such terms of address are now most common, a mature married woman not known as the mother-of-someone is easily identified as unusual. That is not to say that the status of mother-of-someone is unimportant in urban settings—it is, whether or not people use this terminology.

Returning to India in 2010 after an absence of nearly three years with our one-year-old child in tow, Deepak and I began to introduce her to family and friends in Lucknow. I wondered how people would receive her. Because our union crossed many lines of caste, religion, race, and nation, in that sense, bringing this child into existence was an inherently transgressive act in the local moral worlds (Kleinman 1999) of both of our families, whether they thought with their mostly unstated ideals of preserving Kshatriya identity or whiteness. Yet, Anushka's arrival had been eagerly anticipated. So far, people in India have embraced and celebrated her. At times, it feels as though we are the entourage accompanying the celebrity that is our child. That she has been so loved gives me hope for children born and raised into other less conventional families in India and in the United States. At the same time, I am mindful of the influences that our particular situation, our international connections to relatively powerful networks, and our child's highly valued light skin may play in how people in India and the United States see her and us. These privileges are not available to all. And more times than I care to remember, well-meaning women assured me that because Anushka was not a heavy baby, my next baby would surely be a boy.

Soon after we returned to India, we learned that a couple close to our family was expecting a baby. Perhaps because of a previous lost pregnancy, the couple had concealed the pregnancy for many months and only disclosed the impending arrival late in the pregnancy. Since they lived in another city and did not visit often, no one in our home found out until they made the news public in the final trimester. As the conversations and advice about health, delivery, and child-raising began to fly, it became apparent that the couple was desperately hoping for the birth of a boy. Deepak's mother, in particular, answered these wishes with emphatic statements that in this day and age, it doesn't matter whether one has boys or girls, as long as they are healthy. The husband replied that, in any case, he would only have one child, whether it was a boy or a girl. Although ultrasound technology and other biomedical diagnostic tests are available in India, their use for determining the sex of a fetus has been banned because these technologies have been widely utilized to identify and abort female fetuses (Patel 2007a, 2007b).

Combined with long-standing practices of female abandonment and infanticide, these technologies have contributed to enormous gaps in the ratio of male to female children, so much so

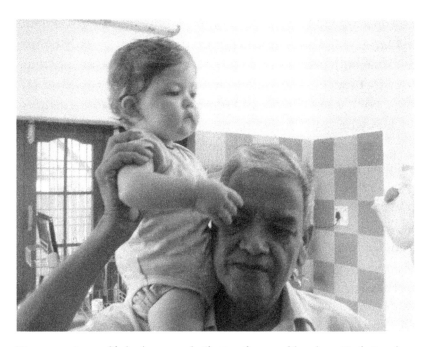

Figure 7.2. A grandfather's care and affection for granddaughter. *Dada ji* and *poti* (paternal grandfather and granddaughter), 2010. (Photo by author.)

that even mentioning the possibility of finding out the sex of the fetus raises eyebrows in polite company. However, that stigma has not ended the practice. Ultrasound technicians can be bribed to pass along the information, and people with sufficient financial resources have been reported to order home sex-determination kits through the internet or to travel to nearby countries where sex determination is allowed. This couple did not, to my knowledge, pursue any of these methods but waited in suspense for the baby's arrival.

The baby was born by caesarean section in a private hospital in Lucknow at full term—a girl. In the midst of comments by others that day that the birth of a boy or girl is irrelevant—although I doubt whether these statements abound at a boy's birth—family members from our home noted the sadness of the wife's side of the family. The maternal grandmother of the new baby, who had no sons, argued back to those who said that boy or girl did not matter, saying that—as was reported to me later—only people who had both boys and girls could feel that there is no difference because they could not understand the lack felt by people without sons. For her, the absence of a son hurt in very mundane matters, such as who could go out to buy milk late at night, never mind long-term concerns about old-age financial security or emotional support. The women of the family, and especially the maternal grandmother, did not hide their desire for a boy or their disappointment at the outcome of this pregnancy. When I asked the husband about whether they would have any more children, he said, "In three years."

As my own daughter grows and shares our lives lived back and forth between India and the United States, always on the move, she has begun asking me questions I find impossible to answer. Her innocence and her insights always give me pause. Sometimes they haunt me. She asks, "Why do those kids outside the mall ask me for money? Why don't their parents give them any?" "Why do the kids in the village only wear underwear?" And in the early-morning space between sleeping and waking, she asks, "Will there ever be a baby in your tummy?"

GLOSSARY

APNA/APNE/APNI (apna/apne/apnī): one's own.

AHAMIYAT (ahamiyat): importance.

AMAANAT (amānat): a trust or charge; see chap. 4.

ASHA (āshā): hope, expectation.

AULAD (aulād): children; see chap. 1.

AYAH (āyah): nursemaid, hospital assistant.

AZAN (azān): call to prayer.

BACCHA (baccā): child, neutral or boy child, depending on context (*bacchi*, girl child; *bacche*, plural male or mixed-gender group).

BADTAMEEZI (badtamīzī): incivility, poor conduct.

BAHU (bahū): daughter-in-law, also young wife or bride.

BAJI (bājī): elder sister, sometimes used as a term of respect with nonrelatives.

BANJH (bānjh): infertile, sterile, barren. Most often used in reference to agricultural land, plants, and women.

BANJHPAN (bānjhpan): sterility, infertility.

BASTI (bastī): a settlement, often used to refer to a makeshift settlement.

BEAULAD/SANTANHIN (beaulād/santānhīn): childless; see chaps. 1 and 4.

BHANJA (bhānja): sister's son, nephew.

BHANJI (bhānji): sister's daughter, niece.

BHABHI (bhābhī): sister-in-law, older brother's wife, sometimes used as a term of respect with nonrelatives.

BHAGVAN (bhagvān): God, used as a general expression.

BHAIYYA (bhaiyya): (informal) brother, friend.

BHATIJA (bhatījā): brother's son, nephew.

BHATIJI (bhatījī): brother's daughter, niece.

BURQA (burqā): a long veil worn over clothes.

CHACHA (cācā): father's younger brother, uncle, sometimes used as a term of respect with nonrelatives.

CHACHI (cācī): father's younger brother's wife, aunt, sometimes used as a term of respect with nonrelatives.

CHIKAN (chikan): style of embroidery famous in Lucknow and surrounding region.

DADA (dādā): father's father, grandfather.

DADI (dādī): father's mother, grandmother.

DAKU/DACOIT (dākū): robber, or one of a band of robbers.

DAMAD (dāmād): son-in-law.

DARGAH (dargāh): Muslim shrine, tomb of a saint.

DEVAR (devar): husband's younger brother.

DEVRANI (devrānī): husband's younger brother's wife.

DHARMA (dharma): right action, duty, virtue, a central concept in Hindu religious and social life.

FITRAT (fitrat): nature, constitution, temperament.

FOETICIDE; feticide: term used in local activism, usually refers to termination of pregnancy based on prenatal sex determination.

GAWA: Guardians and Wards Act of 1890.

GENDA PHOOL (genda phūl): marigold flower.

GHAR (ghar): home, house. Related terms: *ghar chalaana*, to make a home run; *ghar waale*, people of the home; *ghar jamai*, see below.

GHAR JAMAI (ghar jamaī): a live-in son-in-law; see chaps. 1 and 4.

HAMA: Hindu Adoptions and Maintenance Act of 1956.

HIJRA/KINNAR: third sex/gender; see text for additional references.

IMAMBARA (imāmbāṛā): a place where Shi'a Muslims keep religious items used during observances of Muharram. Several prominent Lucknow landmarks are used in this way, and they attract religious visitors, tourists, and others (such as the Bara Imambara and Chota Imambara, "big" and "small").

IVF: in vitro fertilization.

IZZAT (izzat): honor, good name.

JADU (jādū): magic, spell, charm.

JAT/JATI (jāt/jāti): one way of referring to caste identity or affiliation by birth.

JETH (jeth): elder brother.

JETHANI (jethānī): husband's elder brother's wife.

JJA: Juvenile Justice (Care and Protection of Children): Act of 2000, revised in 2006.

KAAM (kām): action, work, business, sexual desire, lovemaking.

KAMZOR (kamzor): weak, feeble.

KHUN (khūn): blood; see chap. 5.

KHUSH KHABRI (khush khabrī): good news.

LUCKNOW/LAKHNAU (lakhnau): capital city of the North Indian state of Uttar Pradesh.

MA BANNA (mā banna): to become a mother.

MAIKA/MAIKE (maikā/maike): natal home, especially home of a married woman's birth family.

MAJBURI (majbūrī): compulsion, powerlessness, helplessness.

MA KI MAMTA (mā kī mamtā): mother's love, affection, tenderness; see chap. 2.

MAMA (māmā): mother's brother.

MAMI (māmī): mother's brother's wife.

MAMTA (mamtā): affection; see chap. 2.

MANDIR (mandir): temple.

MASJID (masjid): a mosque.

MATA (mātā): (formal) mother.

MAZAAR (mazār): a Muslim shrine, tomb.

MUSEEBAT (musībat): a misfortune, disaster, trouble.

NAMASTE (namaste): a greeting at meeting or departure.

NAND (nand): husband's sister, sister-in-law.

NANA (nānā): mother's father, grandfather.

NANI (nānī): mother's mother, grandmother.

NATI (nātī): daughter's son, grandson.

NATIN (nātin): daughter's daughter, granddaughter.

NAWAB (navāb): lord, prince, title of the eighteenth- and nine-teenth-century rulers of Awadh (also spelled Oude), the region in which Lucknow is located.

NAZAR (nazar): sight, glance, gaze, used here in reference to the effects of the evil eye.

NUTFA (nutfa): seed, sperm.

PARCHA (parchā): a piece of paper, a prescription.

PARVARISH (parvarish): fostering, rearing, nurture, support.

PATRILOCAL: a pattern of marriage in which a married couple resides in the male spouse's natal home or community.

POLYANDRY: a form of marriage in which a woman has more than one husband.

POLYGYNY: a form of marriage in which a man has more than one wife.

POTA (pōtā): son's son, grandson.

POTI (pōtī): son's daughter, granddaughter.

PURDAH/PARDA (pardā): curtain, screen, veil; as concept of separation of the sexes, see chap. 1.

QISMAT (qismat): fate, destiny, lot.

RISHTA (rishtā): string, line, connection, relationship.

ROG (rōg): illness, disease, worry, plague.

ROTI (rōṭī): round flatbread made from wheat or other flour.

SAAS/SAASU MA (sās/sāsu mā): husband's mother/wife's mother, mother-in-law.

SADHU (sādhu): an ascetic, a holy man.

SAMAJ (samāj): society or a particular community.

SARI (sāṛī): a sari, iconic dress made of one long piece of cloth, usually six yards long in North India.

SASUR (sasur): husband's father or wife's father, father-in-law.

SASURAL (sasurāl): father-in-law's house or family; see chap. 1.

SAUTELI MA (sautelī mā): father's wife, stepmother.

SHAADI (shādī): wedding, marriage.

SHALWAR KAMEEZ (shalvār kamīz): a form of dress, loose pants and tunic.

SHER (sher): in poetry, a verse or couplet.

TALAQ (talāq): divorce, marital dissolution.

TAMEEZ (tamīz): good sense, courtesy, manners.

TAARIKH/MAHINA (tārīkh/mahīnā): menstrual cycle, menstrual period.

TAAVIZ (tāvīz): an amulet, charm.

TEHZEEB (tahzīb): refinement, culture (in the sense of manners, refined conduct).

UMMID (ummīd): hope, expectation, trust, dependence.

UTTAR PRADESH (uttar pradesh): at the time of research and writing, India's most populous state, located in the north-central Gangetic Plains, with Lucknow as capital.

VANSH (vansh): family line, succession.

ZAKAT (zakāt): portion of property given as alms.

NOTE

Author's definitions, based on relevant context and consulting McGregor ([1993] 1997) and Platts (1977 [1884]).

BIBLIOGRAPHY

Abu-Lughod, Lila. *Do Muslim Women Need Saving?* Cambridge, MA: Harvard University Press, 2013.

———. "Do Muslim Women Really Need Saving?: Anthropological Reflections on Cultural Relativism and Its Others." *American Anthropologist* 104, no. 3 (2002): 783–90.

ACRJ (Asian Communities Reproductive Justice). *A New Vision for Advancing Our Movement for Reproductive Health, Reproductive Rights and Reproductive Justice.* Oakland, CA: ACRJ, 2005. http://strongfamiliesmovement.org/assets/docs/ACRJ-A-New-Vision.pdf.

Ahluwalia, Sanjam. *Reproductive Restraints: Birth Control in India, 1877–1947.* Urbana: University of Illinois Press, 2008.

Ahmad, Imtiaz. "Adoption in India: A Study of Attitudes." *Indian Journal of Social Work* 36, no. 2 (1975): 181–90.

———. "Endogamy and Status Mobility among the Siddiqui Sheikhs of Allahabad, Uttar Pradesh." In *Caste and Social Stratification among Muslims in India,* edited by Imtiaz Ahmad, 171–206. Columbia, MO: South Asia Books, 1978.

———, ed. *Family, Kinship, and Marriage among Muslims in India.* New Delhi: Manohar, 1976.

Alavi, Seema. *Islam and Healing: Loss and Recovery of an Indo-Muslim Medical Tradition, 1600–1900.* London: Palgrave Macmillan, 2008.

Ali, Bharti, and Enakshi Ganguly Thukral. *Combating Child Trafficking: A User's Handbook.* New Delhi: HAQ Centre for Child Rights, 2007.

Anees, Munawar. *Islam and Biological Futures: Ethics, Gender, and Technology*. New York: Mansell, 1989.

Arnold, F., R. A. Bulatao, C. Buripakdi, B. L. Chung, J. T. Fawcett, T. Iritani, S. L. Lee, and T. S. Wu. *The Value of Children: Vol. 1: Introduction and Comparative Analysis*. Honolulu: East-West Population Institute, 1975.

Baabul ki Duaen. Accessed April 10, 2022. https://www.filmyquotes.com /songs/3611.

Bailey, Alison. "Reconceiving Surrogacy: Toward a Reproductive Justice Account of Indian Surrogacy." *Hypatia* 26 (2011): 715–41. https:// doi:10.1111/j.1527–2001.2011.01168.x.

Baird, R. D. *Religion and Law in Independent India*. New Delhi: Manohar, 2005.

Bajpai, R. *Debating Difference: Group Rights and Liberal Democracy in India*. New Delhi; New York: Oxford University Press, 2011.

Bargach, Jamila. *Orphans of Islam: Family, Abandonment, and Secret Adoption in Morocco*. New York: Rowman & Littlefield, 2002.

Barnes, Liberty, and Jasmine Fledderjohann. "Reproductive Justice for the Invisible Infertile: A Critical Examination of Reproductive Surveillance and Stratification." *Sociology Compass* 14 (2020): e12745.

Bateson, Mary Catherine. *Composing a Life*. New York: Atlantic Monthly, 1989.

———. "Participant Observation as a Way of Living." In *Transforming Ethnographic Knowledge*, edited by Rebecca Hardin and Kamari Maxine Clarke, 37–50. Madison: University of Wisconsin Press, 2012.

Behar, Ruth. *The Vulnerable Observer: Anthropology That Breaks Your Heart*. Boston: Beacon, 1996.

Berman, Elise. "Holding On: Adoption, Kinship Tensions, and Pregnancy in the Marshall Islands." *American Anthropologist* 116, no. 3 (2014): 578–590.

Berreman, G. B. "Caste in India and the United States." *American Journal of Sociology* 59, no. 6 (1960): 120–7.

Bhalotra, Sonia, Christine Valente, and Arthur van Soest. "Religion and Childhood Death in India." In *Handbook of Muslims in India: Empirical and Policy Perspectives*, edited by Rakesh Basant and Abusaleh Shariff, 123–64. New Delhi: Oxford, 2009.

Bharadwaj, Aditya. "Biosociality and Biocrossings: Encounters with Assisted Conception and Embryonic Stem Cells in India." In *Biosocialities, Genetics, and the Social Sciences: Making Biologies and Identities*, edited by Sahra Gibbon and Carlos Novas, 98–116. New York: Routledge, 2008.

———. "Conceptions: An Exploration of Infertility and Assisted Conception in India." Diss., University of Bristol, 2001.

———. *Conceptions: Infertility and Procreative Technologies in India.* New York: Berghahn, 2016.

———. "Why Adoption Is Not an Option in India: The Visibility of Infertility, the Secrecy of Donor Insemination, and Other Cultural Complexities." *Social Science and Medicine* 56, no. 9 (2003): 1867–80.

Bharat, S. *Child Adoption: Trends and Emerging Issues.* Bombay: Tata Institute of Social Sciences, 1993.

Bhargava, Vinita. *Adoption in India: Policies and Experiences.* New Delhi: SAGE, 2005.

Bhatia, Shekhar. 2012. "Revealed: How More and More Britons Are Paying Indian Women to Become Surrogate Mothers." *Telegraph*, May 26, 2012.

Bhattacharya, Rinki. *Janani—Mothers, Daughters, Motherhood.* New Delhi: SAGE, 2006.

Billimoria, H. M. *Child Adoption: A Study of Indian Experience.* Himalayan, 1984.

Bledsoe, Caroline. *Contingent Lives: Fertility, Time, and Aging in West Africa.* Chicago: University of Chicago Press, 2002.

Bloom, Shelah S., David Wypij, and Monica Das Gupta. "Dimensions of Women's Autonomy and the Influence on Maternal Health Care Utilization in a North Indian City." *Demography* 38, no. 1 (2001): 67–78.

Bodenhorn, Barbara. "'He Used to Be My Relative': Exploring the Bases of Relatedness among Iñupiat of Northern Alaska." In *Cultures of Relatedness: New Approaches to the Study of Kinship,* edited by Janet Carsten, 128–48. New York: Cambridge University Press, 2000.

Bouhdiba, Abdelwahab. *Sexuality in Islam.* Translated by Alan Sheridan. Boston: Routledge & Kegan Paul, 1985.

Bourdieu, Pierre. *The Logic of Practice.* Stanford: Stanford University Press, 1990.

Browner, Carole H., and Carolyn F. Sargent, eds. *Reproduction, Globalization, and the State: New Theoretical and Ethnographic Perspectives.* Durham, NC: Duke University Press, 2011.

Brunson, Jan. *Planning Families in Nepal: Local and Global Projects of Reproduction.* Brunswick, NJ: Rutgers University Press, 2016.

Bumiller, Elizabeth. *May You Be the Mother of a Hundred Sons: A Journey among the Women of India.* New York: Random House, 1990.

Burke, Jason. 2011. "Census Reveals That 17% of the World Is Indian: Country Closing Gap with China by Adding 181 Million Citizens in Past Decade, Which Is Equivalent to Population of Brazil." *Guardian*, April

1, 2011. Accessed July 16, 2011. http://www.guardian.co.uk/world/2011 /mar/31/census-17-percent-world-indian.

Ceballo, Rosario. "Passion or Data Points? Studying African American Women's Experiences with Infertility." *Qualitative Psychology* 4, no. 3 (2017): 302–14. https://doi-org./10.1037/qup0000079.

Ceballo, Rosario, Erin T. Graham, and Jamie Hart. "Silent and Infertile: An Intersectional Analysis of the Experiences of Socioeconomically Diverse African American Women with Infertility." *Psychology of Women Quarterly* 39, no. 4 (2015): 497–511.

Census of India. 2001. Accessed May 27, 2015. http://censusindia.gov.in /Census_And_You/religion.aspx.

———. 2011. Accessed July 16, 2015. http://www.censusindia.gov.in/2011 -prov-results/data_files/up/Census2011Data%20Sheet-UP.pdf.

———. Central Adoption Resource Authority. Ministry of Women & Child Development, Government of India. Success Stories. Accessed April 13, 2022. http://cara.nic.in/glimpse/sucess_story.html.

Chambers, Brittany D., Helen A. Arega, Silvia E. Arabia, Brianne Taylor, Robyn G. Barron, Brandi Gates, Loretta Scruggs-Leach, Karen A. Scott, and Monica R. McLemore. "Black Women's Perspectives on Structural Racism across the Reproductive Lifespan: A Conceptual Framework for Measurement Development." *Maternal and Child Health Journal* 25 (2021): 402–13. https://doi.org/10.1007/s10995-020-03074-3.

Chandra, Aparna, Mrinal Satish, and the Center for Reproductive Rights. *Securing Reproductive Justice in India: A Casebook*. Delhi: Centre for Constitutional Law, Policy, and Governance, National Law University, 2019.

Chandrachud, D. Y. "In the Matter of Adoption of Payal alias Sharinee Vinay Pathak vs Nil." Indian Adoption Petn No. 31 of 2009, decided September 16, 2009. 2010 (1) AIR Bom R 327:: 2010 AIHC 1846 (BOMBAY HIGH COURT): AIR 2010 (NOC) (Supp) 129 (BOM.), 2009.

Char, Arundhati, Minna Säävälä, and Teija Kulmala. "Mothers-in-Law's Influence on Young Couples' Use of Temporary Contraceptive Methods in Rural Central India." *Reproductive Health Matters* 18, no. 35 (2010): 154–62.

Charsley, Katharine. "Unhappy Husbands: Masculinity and Migration in Transnational Pakistani Marriages." *Journal of the Royal Anthropological Institute* 11, no. 1 (2005): 85–105.

Chase, Susan E., and Mary F. Rogers, eds. *Mothers and Children: Feminist Analyses and Personal Narratives*. New Brunswick, NJ: Rutgers University Press, 2001.

Chopra, Ravi, Amitabh Bachchan, Hema Malini, and Paresh Rawal. *Bagh-ban*. India: B. R. Films, 2003.

Choudhry, U. K. "Traditional Practices of Women from India: Pregnancy, Childbirth, and Newborn Care." *Journal of Obstetric, Gynecologic, & Neonatal Nursing* 26 (1997): 533–39.

Chowdhry, Prem. *Contentious Marriages, Eloping Couples: Gender, Caste, and Patriarchy in Northern India*. New Delhi: Oxford University Press, 2007.

Cohen, Lawrence. "Operability, Bioavailability, and Exception." In *Global Assemblages: Technology, Politics, and Ethics as Anthropological Problems*, edited by Aihwa Ong and Stephen J. Collier, 79–90. Oxford: Blackwell, 2005.

Colen, Shellee. "Like a Mother to Them": Stratified Reproduction and West Indian Childcare Workers and Employers in New York. In *Conceiving the New World Order: The Global Politics of Reproduction*, edited by Faye D. Ginsburg and Rayna Rapp, 78–102. Berkeley: University of California Press, 1995.

Conklin, Beth A., and Lynn M. Morgan. "Babies, Bodies, and Production of Personhood." *Ethos* 24, no. 4 (1996): 657–94.

Crear-Perry, Joia, Rosaly Correa-de-Araujo, Tamara Lewis Johnson, Monica R. McLemore, Elizabeth Neilson, and Maeve Wallace. "Social and Structural Determinants of Health: Inequities in Maternal Health." *Journal of Women's Health* 30, no. 2 (2021): 230–35. https://doi.org.10.1089/jwh.2020.8882.

Cuno, Kenneth M., and Manisha Desai, eds. *Family, Gender, and Law in a Globalizing Middle East and South Asia*. Syracuse, NY: Syracuse University Press, 2009.

Das Gupta, Monica. "Life Course Perspectives on Women's Autonomy and Health Outcomes." *American Anthropologist* 97, no. 3 (1995): 481–91.

———. "Selective Discrimination against Female Children in Rural Punjab, India." *Population and Development Review* 13, no. 1 (1987): 77–100.

DasGupta, Sayantani, and Shamita Das Dasgupta. *Globalization and Transnational Surrogacy in India: Outsourcing Life*. Lanham, MD: Lexington, 2014.

Davis, Dána-Ain. *Reproductive Injustice: Racism, Pregnancy, and Premature Birth*. New York: New York University Press, 2019.

Delaney, Carol. "The Meaning of Paternity and the Virgin Birth Debate." *Man* 21, no. 3 (1986): 494–513.

———. *The Seed and the Soil: Gender and Cosmology in Turkish Village Society*. Berkeley: University of California Press, 1991.

Deomampo, Daisy. "Gendered Geographies of Reproductive Tourism." *Gender & Society* 27, no. 4 (2013): 514–37.

———. *Transnational Reproduction: Race, Kinship, and Commercial Surrogacy in India.* New York: New York University Press, 2016.

Desai, Manisha. "Legal Pluralism versus a Uniform Civil Code: The Continuing Debates in India." In *Family, Gender, and Law in a Globalizing Middle East and South Asia,* edited by Kenneth M. Cuno and Manisha Desai, 65–78. Syracuse: Syracuse University Press, 2009.

Deshpande, Shashi. "Learning to Be a Mother." In *Janani: Mothers, Daughters, Motherhood,* edited by Rinki Bhattacharya, 131–37. New Delhi: SAGE, 2006.

Desjarlais, Robert R. *Body and Emotion: The Aesthetics of Illness and Healing in the Nepal Himalayas.* Philadelphia: University of Pennsylvania Press, 1992.

Diamond, Jared. 2008. "What's Your Consumption Factor?" *New York Times,* January 2, 2008. Accessed June 22, 2021. http://www.nytimes .com/2008/01/02/opinion/02diamond.html?ex=1357016400&en=8d884 753e0aaba6f&ei=5124&partner=permalink&exprod=permalink.

Di Leonardo, Michaela. "The Female World of Cards and Holidays: Women, Families, and the Work of Kinship." *Signs* 12, no. 3 (1987): 440–53.

Dolgin, Janet L. *Defining the Family: Law, Technology, and Reproduction in an Uneasy Age.* New York: New York University Press, 1997.

Dorow, Sara K. *Transnational Adoption: A Cultural Economy of Race, Gender, and Kinship.* New York: New York University Press, 2006.

Douglass, Carrie, ed. *Barren States: The Population "Implosion" in Europe.* New York: Berg, 2005.

Drèze, Jean, and Mamta Murthi. "Fertility, Education, and Development: Evidence from India." *Population and Development Review* 27, no. 1 (2001): 22–63.

Dube, Leela. "Dharti aur Bij." In *Stri ke Lie Jagah* (Hindi), edited by Rajkishore, 50–64. New Delhi: Vani Prakashan, 1994.

Dumont, Louis. *Homo Hierarchicus: The Caste System and Its Implications.* Complete rev. English ed. Chicago: University of Chicago Press, 1967 [1980].

Dyson, Tim, and Mick Moore. "On Kinship Structure, Female Autonomy, and Demographic Behavior in India." *Population and Development Review* 9, no. 1 (1983): 35–60.

Eck, Diana L. *Darśan: Seeing the Divine Image in India.* 3rd ed. New York: Columbia University Press, 1998.

Ehrlich, Paul R. *The Population Bomb*. New York: Ballantine, 1968.

Engineer, Asghar Ali. *Problems of Muslim Women in India*. Bombay: Orient Longman, 1995.

Express News Service. 2010. "Sushmita Can Keep Her Baby." *Express India*, January 14, 2010. Accessed April 12, 2022. http://indianexpress.com /article/cities/mumbai/sushmita-can-keep-her-baby/.

Farmer, Paul. *Infections and Inequalities: The Modern Plagues*. Berkeley: University of California Press, 1999.

Fisher, Michael H., ed. *The Politics of the British Annexation of India, 1757–1857*. Delhi: Oxford University Press, 1993.

Fledderjohann, Jasmine, and Liberty Walther Barnes. "Reimagining Infertility: A Critical Examination of Fertility Norms, Geopolitics and Survey Bias." *Health Policy and Planning* 33 no. 1 (2018): 34–40. https:// doi.org/10.1093/heapol/czx148.

Foucault, Michel. *The History of Sexuality*. Translated by Robert Hurley. New York: Pantheon, 1978.

Frank, Zippi Brand, Zvi Frank, Geraldine Doogue, Uri Akerman, Tal Raviner, and Karni Postel. *Google Baby*. 76 minutes. New York: Filmakers Library, 2009.

Franklin, Sarah. *Embodied Progress: A Cultural Account of Assisted Conception*. New York: Routledge, 1997.

Freed, Ruth S., and Stanley A. Freed. "Beliefs and Practices Resulting in Female Deaths and Fewer Females Than Males in India." *Population and Environment* 10, no. 3 (1989): 144–61.

Gahlot, Deepa. "No Baby, No Cry!" In *Janani: Mothers, Daughters, Motherhood*, edited by Rinki Bhattacharya, 138–45. New Delhi: SAGE, 2006.

Ganguly, Sujata, and Sayeed Unisa. "Trends of Infertility and Childlessness in India: Findings from NFHS Data." *Facts, Views and Vision in ObGyn* 2, no. 2 (2010): 131–38.

Gazette of India. 2015. Government of India, Ministry of Women and Child Development. Part II, section 3, subsection (ii), New Delhi, July 17, 2015.

Geruso, M., and D. Spears. "Sanitation and Health Externalities: Resolving the Muslim Mortality Paradox." *University of Texas at Austin Working Paper*.

Ghosh, Abantika, and Vijaita Singh. 2015. "Census: Hindu Share Dips Below 80%, Muslim Share Grows but Slower." *Indian Express*, January 24, 2015. Accessed May 27, 2015.

Ginsburg, Faye D., and Rayna Rapp. "Introduction: Conceiving the New World Order." In *Conceiving the New World Order: The Global Politics of*

Reproduction, edited by Rayna Rapp and Faye D. Ginsburg, 1–21. Berkeley: University of California Press, 1995.
———. "The Politics of Reproduction." *Annual Review of Anthropology* 20 (1991): 311–43.
Godelier, Maurice. *The Enigma of the Gift.* Oxford: Polity, 1999.
Gogoi, Ranjan J. 2014. Shabnam Hashmi Vs UOI & Ors Writ Petition (Civil) No. 470 of 2005 IN THE SUPREME COURT OF INDIA CIVIL ORIGINAL JURISDICTION WRIT PETITION (CIVIL) NO. 470 OF 2005 SHABNAM HASHMI . . . PETITIONER(S) VERSUS UNION OF INDIA & ORS. . . . RESPONDENT (S) JUDGMENT.
Government of India Ministry of Health and Family Welfare. 2021. *Maternal Mortality Reports.* 2010–2012. Accessed August 18, 2015. http://pib .nic.in/newsite/PrintRelease.aspx?relid=103446. 2016–18. Accessed June 4, 2021. https://www.pib.gov.in/PressReleasePage.aspx?PRID=1697441.
Greenhalgh, Susan. *Cultivating Global Citizens: Population in the Rise of China.* Cambridge: Harvard University Press, 2010.
———. *Just One Child: Science and Policy in Deng's China.* Berkeley: University of California Press, 2008.
Greenhalgh, Susan, and Edward A. Winckler. *Governing China's Population: From Leninist to Neoliberal Politics.* Stanford, CA: Stanford University Press, 2005.
Gregory, C. A. *Savage Money: The Anthropology and Politics of Commodity Exchange.* Amsterdam: Harwood Academic, 1997.
Greil, Arthur L. *Not Yet Pregnant: Infertile Couples in Contemporary America.* New Brunswick, NJ: Rutgers University Press, 1991.
Greil, Arthur L., and Julia McQuillan. "'Trying' Times: Medicalization, Intent, and Ambiguity in the Definition of Infertility." *Medical Anthropology Quarterly* 24, no. 2 (2010): 137–56.
Grey, Daniel J. R. "She Gets the Taunts and Bears the Blame: Infertility in Contemporary India." In *The Palgrave Handbook of Infertility in History: Approaches, Contexts and Perspectives,* edited by Gayle Davis and Tracey Loughran, 241–62. London: Palgrave Macmillan, 2017.
Gupta, Aditi, and Tuhin Paul. *Menstrupedia Comic: The Friendly Guide to Periods for Girls.* India: Menstrupedia, 2014.
Gupta, Akhil. *Red Tape: Bureaucracy, Structural Violence, and Poverty in India.* Durham, NC: Duke University Press, 2012.
Gupta, Charu. *Sexuality, Obscenity, Community: Women, Muslims, and the Hindu Public in Colonial India.* New Delhi: Permanent Black, 2001.
Gupta, Jayoti. "Land, Dowry, Labour: Women in the Changing Economy of Midnapur." *Social Scientist* 21, nos. 9/11 (1993): 74–90.

Haimowitz, Rebecca, and Vaishali Sinha. *Made in India: A Film about Surrogacy*. 97 minutes. New York: Women Make Movies, 2010.

Haraway, Donna. "Situated Knowledges: The Science Question in Feminism and the Privilege of Partial Perspective." *Feminist Studies* 14, no. 3 (1988): 575–99. https://doi.org.10.2307/3178066.

Hartmann, Betsy. *Reproductive Rights and Wrongs: The Global Politics of Population Control and Reproductive Choice*. New York: Harper & Row, 1987.

Hasan, Zoya, and Ritu Menon. *The Diversity of Muslim Women's Lives in India*. New Brunswick, NJ: Rutgers University Press, 2005.

———. *Unequal Citizens: A Study of Muslim Women in India*. New Delhi: Oxford University Press, 2004.

Haworth, Abigail. "Surrogate Mothers: Womb for Rent." *Marie Claire*, July 29, 2007. Accessed January 30, 2014. http://www.marieclaire.com /world-reports/news/surrogate-mothers-india.

Heitmeyer, Carolyn, and Maya Unnithan. "Bodily Rights and Collective Claims: The Work of Legal Activists in Interpreting Reproductive and Maternal Rights in India." *Journal of the Royal Anthropological Institute* 21 (2015): 374–90. doi.10.1111/1467-9655.12211.

Heng, Geraldine, and Janadas Devan. "State Fatherhood: The Politics of Nationalism, Sexuality, and Race in Singapore." In *Nationalisms and Sexualities*, edited by Andrew Parker, Mary Russo, Doris Sommer, and Patricia Yaeger, 344–64. New York: Routledge, 1992.

Hodgson, Marshall G. S. *The Venture of Islam, Vol 1*. Chicago: University of Chicago Press, 1974.

Holt, Sarah, J. Mow, C. Schmidt, J. Olicker, and O. Platt. *World in the Balance*. Boston: WGBH Educational Foundation, 2004.

Howell, Signe Lise. *The Kinning of Foreigners: Transnational Adoption in a Global Perspective*. Berghahn, 2006.

———. "Self-Conscious Kinship: Some Contested Values in Norwegian Transnational Adoption." In *Relative Values: Reconfiguring Kinship Studies*, edited by Sarah Franklin and Susan McKinnon, 203–23. Durham, NC: Duke University Press, 2001.

Husain, Sheikh Abrar. *Marriage Customs among Muslims in India: A Sociological Study of the Shi'a Marriage Customs*. New Delhi: Sterling, 1976.

In-Country Research and Data Collection on Forced Labor and Child Labor in the Production of Goods: India. Washington, DC: US Dept. of Labor, Bureau of International Labor Affairs, Office of Child Labor, Forced Labor, and Human Trafficking, 2009.

Indian Council of Medical Research (ICMR). *National Guidelines for Accreditation, Supervision and Regulation of ART Clinics in India.* New Delhi: Ministry of Health and Family Welfare, Government of India, 2005.

Indian Express Online. 2014. "Ashish Bose, Who Coined Bimaru, Dies at 84." ENS Economic Bureau, April 8, 2014.

Indian Express. 2015. "Census: Hindu Share Dips Below 80%, Muslim Share Grows but Slower," January 24, 2015 Accessed May 27, 2015. http://indianexpress.com/article/india/india-others/census-hindu -share-dips-below-80-muslim-share-grows-but-slower/.

Inhorn, Marcia C. *Cosmopolitan Conceptions: IVF Sojourns in Global Dubai.* Durham, NC: Duke University Press, 2015.

———. "Defining Women's Health: A Dozen Messages from More Than 150 Ethnographies." *Medical Anthropology Quarterly* 20, no. 3 (2008): 345–78.

———. "'He Won't Be My Son': Middle Eastern Men's Discourses of Adoption and Gamete Donation." *Medical Anthropology Quarterly* 20, no. 1 (2006): 94–120.

———. *Infertility and Patriarchy: The Cultural Politics of Family Life in Egypt.* Philadelphia: University of Pennsylvania Press, 1996.

———. *Local Babies, Global Science: Gender, Religion and In Vitro Fertilization in Egypt.* New York: Routledge, 2003.

———. *Quest for Conception: Gender, Infertility, and Egyptian Medical Traditions.* Philadelphia: University of Pennsylvania Press, 1994.

———, ed. *Reproductive Disruptions: Gender, Technology, and Biopolitics in the New Millennium.* Oxford: Berghahn, 2007.

Inhorn, Marcia C., Rosario Ceballo, and Robert Nachtigall. "Marginalized, Invisible and Unwanted: American Minority Struggles with Infertility and Assisted Conception." In *Marginalized Reproduction: Ethnicity, Infertility and Reproductive Technologies,* edited by Lorraine Culley, Nicky Hudson, and Floor van Rooij, 181–98. Sterling, VA: Earthscan, 2009.

Inhorn, Marcia C., and Pankaj Shrivastav. "Globalization and Reproductive Tourism in the United Arab Emirates." *Asia-Pacific Journal of Public Health* 22, suppl. 3 (2010): 68S–74S.

International Institute for Population Sciences (IIPS) and ORC Macro. *National Family Health Survey (NFHS-2), India, 1998–99: Uttar Pradesh.* Mumbai: IIPS, 2001.

Islam, Shamsul. "Kyunki Aurtein Tumhari Kheti Hain." In *Stri ke Lie Jagah* (Hindi), edited by Rajkishore, 65–71. New Delhi: Vani Prakashan, 1994.

Iyer, Sriya. *Demography and Religion in India*. New Delhi: Oxford University Press, 2002.

Jain, Bharti. 2015. "Muslim Population Grows 24%, Slower Than Previous Decade." *Times of India*, January 22, 2015. Accessed October 21, 2017. https://timesofindia.indiatimes.com/india/Muslimpopulation-grows-24-slower-than-previous-decade/articleshow/45972687.cms.

Jaitly, Jaya. 2007. "Counting Heads, Missing the Picture." *New Indian Express*, June 2, 2007. Accessed September 17, 2015. http://archive.indianexpress.com/news/counting-heads-missing-the-picture/32470/.

Jasanoff, Sheila, ed. *States of Knowledge: The Co-Production of Science and Social Order*. New York: Routledge, 2004.

Jauregui, Beatrice. "Provisional Agency in Northern India: *Jugaad* and Legitimation of Corruption." *American Ethnologist* 41 no. 1 (2014): 76–91.

Jeffery, Patricia, and Roger Jeffery. *Confronting Saffron Demography: Religion, Fertility, and Women's Status in India*. New Delhi: Three Essays Collective, 2006.

———. *Don't Marry Me to a Plowman!: Women's Everyday Lives in Rural North India*. Boulder, CO: Westview, 1996.

———. "Only When the Boat Has Started Sinking: A Maternal Death in Rural North India." *Social Science & Medicine*, 2010. https://doi.org.10.1016/j.socscimed.2010.05.002.

———. "'We Five, Our Twenty-Five': Myths of Population Out of Control in Contemporary India." In *New Horizons in Medical Anthropology: Essays in Honor of Charles Leslie*, edited by Mark Nichter and Margaret Lock, 172–99. New York: Routledge, 2002.

Jeffery, Patricia, Roger Jeffery, and Andrew Lyon. *Labour Pains and Labour Power: Women and Childbearing in India*. New Jersey: Zed, 1989.

Jeffery, Roger, and Patricia Jeffery. *Population, Gender, and Politics: Demographic Change in Rural North India*. Cambridge: Cambridge University Press, 1997.

Jejeebhoy, Shireen. "Addressing Women's Reproductive Health Needs: Priorities for the Family Welfare Programme." *Economic & Political Weekly* 32, nos. 9/10 (1997): 475–84.

———. "Infertility in India—Levels, Patterns, and Consequences: Priorities for Social Science Research." *Journal of Family Welfare* 44, no. 2 (1998): 15–24.

Jejeebhoy, Shireen J., and Zeba A. Sathar. "Women's Autonomy in India and Pakistan: The Influence of Religion and Region." *Population and Development Review* 27, no. 4 (2001): 687–712.

Jerosch, Rainer. *The Rani of Jhansi, Rebel against Will: A Biography of the Legendary Indian Freedom Fighter in the Mutiny of 1857–1858*. Delhi: Aakar, 2007.

Johnson, Katherine M., Arthur L. Greil, Karina M. Shreffler, and Julia McQuillan. "Fertility and Infertility: Toward an Integrative Research Agenda." *Population Research and Policy Review* 37 (2018): 641–66.

Johnson-Hanks, Jennifer. "On the Limits of Life Stages in Ethnography: Toward a Theory of Vital Conjunctures." *American Anthropologist* 104, no. 3 (2002): 865–80.

———. *Uncertain Honor: Modern Motherhood in an African Crisis*. Chicago: University of Chicago Press, 2006.

Jolly, Margaret. "Introduction: Embodied States—Familial and National Genealogies in Asia and the Pacific." In *Borders of Being: Citizenship, Fertility, and Sexuality in Asia and the Pacific*, edited by Margaret Jolly and Kalpana Ram, 1–35. Ann Arbor: University of Michigan Press, 2001.

Joshi, A. P., M. D. Srinivas, and J. K. Bajaj. *Religious Demography of India*. Chennai, India: Centre for Policy Studies, 2003.

Kahn, Susan. *Reproducing Jews: A Cultural Account of Assisted Conception in Israel*. Durham, NC: Duke University Press, 2000.

Kakar, Sudhir. *The Inner World: A Psycho-Analytic Study of Childhood and Society in India*. Delhi: Oxford University Press, 1978.

Kanaaneh, Rhoda Ann. *Birthing the Nation: Strategies of Palestinian Women in Israel*. Berkeley: University of California Press, 2002.

Kapoor R., P. Kapoor, and N. Dutt. *Awara*. London: Yash Raj Films, 2000 [original release 1951].

Karanth, G. K. "Feeding the Needy Student: Auto-Ethnographic Reflections from South India." *Food, Culture, & Society* 17, no. 3 (2014): 417–32. https://doi.org.10.2752/175174414X13948130848421.

Karve, Irawati. "The Kinship Map of India." In *Family, Kinship, and Marriage in India*, edited by Patricia Uberoi, 50–73. Delhi: Oxford University Press, 1994 [1953].

Khan, M. E. *Family Planning among Muslims in India: A Study of the Reproductive Behavior of Muslims in an Urban Setting*. New Delhi: Manohar, 1979.

Khan, Nasiruddin Haider. *Challenging Myths and Misconceptions: Communicating Women's Rights in Islam*. Health and Population Innovation Fellowship Program. New Delhi: Population Council, 2010.

Khare, R. S. *Caste, Hierarchy, and Individualism: Indian Critiques of Louis Dumont's Contributions*. New Delhi: Oxford University Press, 2006.

———. "Dava, Daktar, and Dua: Anthropology of Practiced Medicine in India." *Social Science and Medicine* 43, no. 5 (1996): 837–48.

———. "From Kanya to Mata: Aspects of the Cultural Language of Kinship in Northern India." In *Concepts of Person: Kinship, Caste, and Marriage in India*, edited by Ákos Östör, Lina Fruzzetti, and Steve Barnett, 143–71. Cambridge, MA: Harvard University Press, 1982.

———. "The Other's Double. The Anthropologist's Bracketed Self: Notes on Cultural Representation and Privileged Discourse." *New Literary History* 23, no. 1 (1992): 1–23.

———. "The *Unch-Nich* Challenge in Life: Changing Locations, Forces, and Meanings." In *Caste in Life: Experiencing Inequalities*, edited by D. Shyam Babu and R. S. Khare, 20–32. New Delhi: Pearson, 2011.

Kleinman, Arthur. "Experience and Its Moral Modes: Culture, Human Conditions, and Disorder." *Tanner Lectures on Human Values* 20 (1999): 357–420.

Kligman, Gail. *The Politics of Duplicity: Controlling Reproduction in Ceausescu's Romania*. Berkeley: University of California Press, 1998.

Kopf, Dan, and Preeti Varathan. 2017. "If Uttar Pradesh Were a Country." *Quartz India*, October 11, 2017. Accessed June 23, 2021. https://qz.com/india/1094942/if-uttar-pradesh-were-a-country-where-would-it-rank-by-size-wealth-and-other-measures/.

Krause, Elizabeth L. *A Crisis of Births: Population Politics and Family-Making in Italy*. Belmont, CA: Wadsworth, 2005.

Krause, Elizabeth L., and Milena Marchesi. "Fertility Politics as 'Social Viagra': Reproducing Boundaries, Social Cohesion, and Modernity in Italy." *American Anthropologist* 109, no. 2 (2007): 350–62.

Lamb, Sarah. *White Saris and Sweet Mangoes: Aging, Gender, and Body in North India*. Berkeley: University of California Press, 2000.

Layne, Linda L. *Motherhood Lost: A Feminist Account of Pregnancy Loss in America*. New York: Routledge, 2003.

Lebra-Chapman, Joyce. *The Rani of Jhansi: A Study in Female Heroism in India*. Honolulu: University of Hawaii Press, 1986.

Leinaweaver, Jessaca. *The Circulation of Children: Kinship, Adoption, and Morality in Andean Peru*. Durham, NC: Duke University Press, 2008.

———. "On Moving Children: The Social Implications of Andean Child Circulation." *American Ethnologist* 34, no. 1 (2007): 163–80.

Llewellyn-Jones, Rosie. *A Fatal Friendship: The Nawabs, the British, and the City of Lucknow*. New York: Oxford University Press, 1985.

Lobo, Aloma, and Jayapriya Vasudevan. *The Penguin Guide to Adoption in India*. New Delhi: Penguin, 2002.

Lulla, Sunil, John Abraham, Shoojit Sircar, Juhi Chaturvedi, Annu Kapoor, Ayushman Khurrana, Yaami Gautam, and Dolly Ahluwalia. *Vicky Donor.* Mumbai: Eros International, 2012.

Luna, Zakiya. "Black Celebrities, Reproductive Justice and Queering Family: An Exploration." *Reproductive Biomedicine and Society Online* 7 (2018): 91–100.

———. *Reproductive Rights as Human Rights: Women of Color and the Fight for Reproductive Justice.* New York: New York University Press, 2020.

Luna, Zakiya, and Kristin Luker. "Reproductive Justice." *Annual Review of Law and Social Science* 9 (2013): 327–52.

Maheshwary, Ram, Manoj Kumar, Waheeda Rehman, Raaj Kumar, Balraj Sahni Mehmood, and Jairai Shashikala. *Neel Kamal [Blue Lotus].* Sacramento, CA: Digital Entertainment, Inc. [1968] 1999.

Majumdar, Anindita. *Transnational Commercial Surrogacy and the (Un)making of Kin in India.* New Delhi: Oxford University Press, 2018.

———. "Transnational Surrogacy: The 'Public' Selection of Selective Discourse." *Economic & Political Weekly* 48, nos. 45/46 (2013): 24–27.

Maloney, Clarence. "India: Don't Say 'Pretty Baby' Lest You Zap It with Your Eye—The Evil Eye in South Asia." In *The Evil Eye,* edited by Clarence Maloney, 102–48. New York: Columbia University Press, 1976.

Mandelbaum, David G. *Human Fertility in India: Social Components and Policy Perspectives.* Berkeley: University of California Press, 1974.

———. *Women's Seclusion and Men's Honor: Sex Roles in North India, Bangladesh, and Pakistan.* Tucson: University of Arizona Press, 1988.

Marre, Diana, and Laura Briggs. *International Adoption: Global Inequalities and the Circulation of Children.* New York: New York University Press, 2009.

Martin, Emily. *The Woman in the Body: A Cultural Analysis of Reproduction.* Boston: Beacon, 1987.

Mayo, Katherine. *Mother India.* New York: Harcourt, Brace, 1927.

McGregor, R. S., ed. *The Oxford Hindi-English Dictionary.* New Delhi: Oxford University Press, [1993] 1997.

McKinnon, Susan. "On Kinship and Marriage: A Critique of the Genetic and Gender Calculus of Evolutionary Psychology." In *Complexities: Beyond Nature and Nurture,* edited by Susan McKinnon and Sydel Silverman, 106–31. Chicago: University of Chicago Press, 2005.

McLemore, Monica R., Ifeyinwa Asiodu, Joia Crear-Perry, Dána-Ain Davis, Michelle Drew, Rachel R. Hardeman, Dara D. Mendez, Lynn Roberts, and Karen A. Scott. "Race, Research, and Women's Health:

Best Practice Guidelines for Investigators." *Obstetrics and Gynecology* 134, no. 2 (2019): 422–23.

Mehra, Rakeysh Omprakash, Ronnie Screwvala, Prasoon Joshi, Kamlesh Pandey, Waheeda Rehman, Tanvi Azmi, Abhishek Bachchan, et al. *Dilli-6 Delhi-6*. Marina del Ray, CA: UTV Home Entertainment, 2009.

Mishra, Manjari. 2007. "A Desire to Adopt Child Faces Hurdle." *Times of India*, July 15 2007, Lucknow edition.

Mishra, Ramesh C., Boris Mayer, Gisella Trommsdorff, Isabelle Albert, and Beate Schwarz. "The Value of Children in Urban and Rural India: Cultural Background and Empirical Results." In *The Value of Children in Cross-Cultural Perspective: Case Studies from Eight Societies*, edited by Gisela Trommsdorff and Bernhard Nauck, 143–70. Lengerich: Pabst Science, 2005.

Modell, Judith Schachter. *Kinship with Strangers: Adoption and Interpretations of Kinship in American Culture*. Berkeley: University of California Press, 1994.

———. "Rights to the Children: Foster Care and Social Reproduction in Hawaii." In *Reproducing Reproduction: Kinship, Power, and Technological Innovation*, edited by Sarah Franklin and Helena Ragoné, 156–72. Philadelphia: University of Pennsylvania Press, 1998.

———. *A Sealed and Secret Kinship: The Culture of Policies and Practices in American Adoption*. Houndmills, Basingstoke, Hampshire, UK: Palgrave, 2002.

Mody, Perveez. *The Intimate State: Love-Marriage and the Law in Delhi*. New Delhi: Routledge, 2008.

Mohan, Surendra. *Awadh under the Nawabs: Politics, Culture and Communal Relations, 1722–1856*. Delhi: Manohar, 1997.

Mohanty, Jayashree, Jaejin Ahn, and Srinivasan Chokkanathan. "Adoption Disclosure: Experiences of Indian Domestic Adoptive Parents." *Child and Family Social Work* (2014). https://doi.org.10.1111/cfs.12175.

Moosa, Ebrahim. "*Shari'at* Governance in Colonial and Post-Colonial India." In *Islam in South Asia in Practice*, edited by Barbara Daly Metcalf, 317–25. Princeton, NJ: Princeton University Press, 2009.

Mukherjee, Rudrangshu. *Awadh in Revolt 1857–58: A Study of Popular Resistance*. Delhi: Oxford University Press, 1984.

Mulgaonkar, Veena B. "Childless Couples in the Slums of Mumbai: An Interdisciplinary Study." *Asia-Pacific Population Journal* 16, no. 2 (2001): 141–60.

Nag, Moni. "Beliefs and Practices about Food during Pregnancy: Implications for Maternal Nutrition." *Economic & Political Weekly* 29, no. 37 (1994): 2427–38.

Nanda, Serena. *Neither Man nor Woman: The Hijras of India.* Belmont, CA: Wadsworth, 1990.

Nandagiri, Rishita. "Nirdhāra: A Multimethod Study of Women's Abortion Trajectories in Karnataka, India." PhD thesis, London School of Economics and Political Science, 2019.

National Family Health Survey, India. International Institute for Population Sciences. Key Findings from NFHS-3. Accessed April 13, 2022.

Nichter, M. "Idioms of Distress: Alternatives in the Expression of Psychosocial Distress: A Case Study from South India." *Culture, Medicine, and Psychiatry* 5 (1981): 379–408.

Padmanabhan, Chitra. "Muslims Up, Hindus Down: The Perils of Reading the Census as Sensex." *The Wire,* vol. 27, August 2015. Accessed December 6, 2018. https://science.thewire.in/health /the-perils-of-reading-the-census-as-a-sensex-of-religion/.

Pande, Amrita. "'At Least I Am Not Sleeping with Anyone': Resisting the Stigma of Commercial Surrogacy in India." Special issue, "Re-inventing Mothers." *Feminist Studies* 36, no. 2 (2010): 292–312.

———. "'It May Be Her Eggs but It's My Blood': Surrogates and Everyday Forms of Kinship in India." *Qualitative Sociology* 32, no. 4 (2009a): 379–97.

———. "Not an 'Angel,' Not a 'Whore': Surrogates as 'Dirty' Workers in India." *Indian Journal of Gender Studies* 16, no. 2 (2009b): 141–73.

———. "Revisiting Surrogacy in India: Domino Effects of the Ban." *Journal of Gender Studies* 30, no. 4 (2021): 395–405. doi.10.1080/09589236 .2020.1830044.

———. *Wombs in Labor: Transnational Commercial Surrogacy in India.* New York: Columbia University Press, 2014.

Papanek, Hanna, and Gail Minault, eds. *Separate Worlds: Studies of Purdah in South Asia.* New Delhi: Chanakya, 1982.

Parry, Jonathan P. *Death in Banaras.* Cambridge: Cambridge University Press, 1994.

Partners in Health. Twitter, 2012. Accessed September 28, 2015. https:// twitter.com/pih/status/224177665551237121.

Patel, Tulsi. *Fertility Behavior: Population and Society in a Rajasthan Village.* Delhi: Oxford University Press, 1994.

———. "Introduction: Gender Relations, NRTs and Female Foeticide in India." In *Sex-Selective Abortion in India: Gender, Society and New*

Reproductive Technologies, edited by Tulsi Patel, 27–58. New Delhi: SAGE, 2007a.

———, ed. *Sex-Selective Abortion in India: Gender, Society and New Reproductive Technologies*. New Delhi: SAGE, 2007b.

Paxson, Heather. *Making Modern Mothers: Ethics and Family Planning in Modern Greece*. Berkeley: University of California Press, 2004.

Pinto, Sarah. "Casting Desire: Reproduction, Loss, and Subjectivity in Rural North India." Diss., Princeton University, 2003.

———. "Development without Institutions: Ersatz Medicine and the Politics of Everyday Life in Rural North India." *Cultural Anthropology* 19, no. 3 (2004): 337–64.

———. *Where There Is No Midwife: Birth and Loss in Rural India*. New York: Berghahn, 2008.

Philipose, Pamela, and Mukul Kesavan. "The #MeToo Movement." *Indian Journal of Gender Studies* 26, nos. 1/2 (2019): 207–14. https://doi .org/10.1177/0971521518812288.

Platts, John T. *A Dictionary of Urdu, Classical Hindi, and English*. New Delhi: Munshiram Manoharlal, 1977 [1884].

Population Council [Friday Okonofua and Bishakha Datta]. "'What About Us?' Bringing Infertility into Reproductive Health Care." *Quality/ Calidad/Qualité*, no. 13 (2002).

Population Reference Bureau. 2015. Data Finder, Infant Mortality Rate (infant deaths per 1,000 live births), 1970 and 2013. Accessed April 14, 2022. https://interactives.prb.org/wpds/2014/index.html.

———. 2020. *2020 World Population Data Sheet*. Accessed May 29, 2021. https://interactives.prb.org/2020-wpds/download-files/.

Pradhan, Karan. "Religion in Numbers: What 2011 Census Reveals about India's Communities." *FirstPost*, August 27, 2015. Accessed October 12, 2015. http://www.firstpost.com/politics/religion-innumbers-what-the -2011-census-revealed-about-trends-across-indias-communities-2408740 .html.

Pradhana, Gauri. *Back Home from Brothels: A Case Study of the Victims of Commercial Sexual Exploitation and Trafficking across Nepal-India Border*. 3rd ed. Kathmandu: Child Workers in Nepal Concerned Center, 1997.

Qureshi, Bashir Ahmad. *Standard Twentieth Century Dictionary: Urdu into English*. Reviewed by Abdul Haq. Delhi: Educational Publishing House, 1999.

Rabinowiz, Abby. "The Surrogacy Cycle." *Virginia Quarterly Review* 92, no. 2 (2016). Accessed April 20, 2016. http://www.vqronline.org /reporting-articles/2016/03/surrogacy-cycle.

Ragoné, Heléne, and France Winddance Twine, eds. *Ideologies and Technologies of Motherhood: Race, Class, Sexuality, Nationalism.* New York:
Routledge, 2000.

Raheja, Gloria Goodwin. *The Poison in the Gift: Ritual, Prestation, and the
Dominant Caste in a North Indian Village.* Chicago: University of Chicago Press, 1988.

Rajan, Rajeshwari Sundar. *The Scandal of the State: Women, Law, and Citizenship in Postcolonial India.* Durham, NC: Duke University Press, 2003.

Ram, Kalpana. "Rationalizing Fecund Bodies: Family Planning Policy and
the Modern Indian Nation State." In Margaret Jolly and Kalpana Ram,
eds. *Borders of Being: Citizenship, Fertility, and Sexuality in Asia and the
Pacific.* Ann Arbor: University of Michigan Press, 2001.

Ramberg, Lucinda. *Given to the Goddess: South Indian Devadasis and the
Sexuality of Religion.* Durham, NC: Duke University Press, 2014.

Rao, Mohan. *From Population Control to Reproductive Health: Malthusian
Arithmetic.* New Delhi: SAGE, 2004.

Rapp, Rayna. "Moral Pioneers: Women, Men and Fetuses on a Frontier
of Reproductive Technology." In *Embryos, Ethics, and Women's Rights:
Exploring the New Reproductive Technologies,* edited by Elaine Hoffman
Baruch, Amadeo F. D'Adamo Jr., and Joni Seager, 101–16. New York:
Haworth, 1988.

———. *Testing Women, Testing the Fetus: The Social Impact of Amniocentesis in America.* New York: Routledge, 1999.

Ray, Satyajit. *Shatranj ke Khilari.* [*The Chess Players.*] Screenplay by
Satyajit Ray. Directed by Satyajit Ray. Performed by Sanjeev Kumar,
Saeed Jaffrey, Amjad Khan, Richard Attenborough, and Shabana Azmi.
India: Devki Chitra Productions, 1977.

Reddy, Gayatri. *With Respect to Sex: Negotiating Hijra Identity in South
India.* Chicago: University of Chicago Press, 2005.

Riessman, Catherine Kohler. "Positioning Gender Identity in Narratives
of Infertility: South Indian Women's Lives in Context." In *Infertility
around the Globe: New Thinking on Childlessness, Gender, and Reproduction,* edited by Marcia C. Inhorn and Frank van Balen, 152–70. Berkeley:
University of California Press, 2002.

Riley, Nancy E. "Stratified Reproduction." In *International Handbook on
Gender and Demographic Processes,* edited by Nancy E. Riley and Jan
Brunson, 117–38. Dordrecht, Netherlands: Springer, 2018.

Riley, Nancy E., and James McCarthy. *Demography in the Age of the
Postmodern.* Cambridge: Cambridge University Press, 2003.

Riley, Nancy E., and Jan Brunson. "Introduction." In *International Handbook on Gender and Demographic Processes*, edited by Nancy E. Riley and Jan Brunson, 1–11. Dordrecht, Netherlands: Springer, 2018.

Roberts, Dorothy E. *Killing the Black Body: Race, Reproduction, and the Meaning of Liberty*. New York: Pantheon, 1997.

———. *Shattered Bonds: The Color of Child Welfare*. New York: Basic Books, 2002.

Ross, Loretta. "Understanding Reproductive Justice: Transforming the Pro-Choice Movement." *Off Our Backs* 36, no. 4 (2006): 14–19. https://doi.org.10.2307/20838711.

Ross, Loretta J., Lynn Roberts, Erika Derkas, Whitney Peoples, and Pamela Bridgewater Toure, eds. *Radical Reproductive Justice: Foundations, Theory, Practice, Critique*. New York: Feminist Press, 2017.

Ross, Loretta J., and Rickie Solinger. *Reproductive Justice: An Introduction*. Oakland: University of California Press, 2017.

Rothman, Barbara Katz. *Recreating Motherhood: Ideology and Technology in a Patriarchal Society*. New York: Norton, 1990.

Rozario, M. Rita. *Trafficking in Women and Children in India: Sexual Exploitation and Sale*. New Delhi: Uppal Publishing House for William Carey Women's Programme, 1988.

Rudrappa, Sharmila. *Discounted Life: The Price of Global Surrogacy in India*. New York: New York University Press, 2015.

———. "India Outlawed Commercial Surrogacy—Clinics Are Finding Loopholes." *The Conversation*, October 23, 2017. Accessed June 18, 2021. https://theconversation.com/india-outlawed-commercial-surrogacy -clinics-are-finding-loopholes-81784.

Säävälä, Minna. "Understanding the Prevalence of Female Sterilization in Rural South India." *Studies in Family Planning* 30, no. 4 (1999): 288–301.

Sachar, R. *Social, Economic and Educational Status of the Muslim Community in India*. New Delhi: Cabinet Secretariat, Government of India, 2006.

Sachedina, Abdulaziz. *Islamic Biomedical Ethics: Principles and Application*. New York: Oxford University Press, 2009.

Sadanah, Vijay, dir. *Aulad*. Produced by Chandar Sadanah. Performed by Jeetendra, Sridevi, Jayapradha, Saeed Jaffrey, Asrani, and Vinod Mehra. Bombay: Shiva Video, 1987.

Sama Resource Group for Women and Health. *Birthing a Market: A Study on Commercial Surrogacy*, 2012. India: Sama Resource Group for Women and Health. Accessed November 3, 2013. https://www.samawomenshealth .org/publication/birthing-market-_commercial-surrogacy-india/.

———. *Constructing Conceptions: The Mapping of Assisted Reproductive Technologies in India*, 2010. India: Sama Resource Group for Women and Health.

Sample Registration System. Compendium of India's Fertility and Mortality Indicators, 1971–2013. Accessed April 10, 2022. https://censusindia.gov.in/vital_statistics/Compendium/Srs_data.html

Sample Registration System Statistical Report 2018. Accessed May 27, 2021. https://censusindia.gov.in/vital_statistics/SRS_Reports_2018.html.

Sandelowski, Margarete. *With Child in Mind: Studies of the Personal Encounter with Infertility*. Philadelphia: University of Pennsylvania Press, 1993.

Sandelowski, Margarete, and Sheryl de Lacey. "The Uses of a 'Disease': Infertility as Rhetorical Vehicle." In *Infertility around the Globe: New Thinking on Childlessness, Gender, and Reproductive Technologies*, edited by Frank van Balen and Marcia Inhorn, 33–51. Berkeley: University of California Press, 2002.

Saravanan, Sheela. *A Transnational Feminist View of Surrogacy Biomarkets in India*. Singapore: Springer, 2018.

Scheper-Hughes, Nancy. *Death without Weeping: The Violence of Everyday Life in Brazil*. Berkeley: University of California Press, 1992.

Schiavocampo, Mara. "More and More Couples Finding Surrogates in India." *The Today Show*, February 20, 2008. Accessed December 19, 2013. http://www.today.com/id/23252624#.UouOkuLlfMg.

Scott, Karen A. "The Rise of Black Feminist Intellectual Thought and Political Activism in Perinatal Quality Improvement: A Righteous Rage about Racism, Resistance, Resilience, and Rigor." *Feminist Anthropology* 2 (2021): 155–60. https://doi.org.10.1002/fea2.12045.

Scott, Karen A., Laura Britton, and Monica R. McLemore. "The Ethics of Perinatal Care for Black Women: Dismantling the Structural Racism in 'Mother Blame' Narratives." *Journal of Perinatal & Neonatal Nursing* 33, no. 2 (2019): 108–15.

Sen, Amartya. *Development as Freedom*. 1st. ed. New York: Knopf, 1999.

———. "India's Women: The Mixed Truth." *New York Review of Books*, October 10, 2013. Accessed September 17, 2015. http://www.nybooks.com/articles/archives/2013/oct/10/indias-women-mixed-truth/.

———. "More Than 100 Million Women Are Missing." *New York Review of Books*, December 20, 1990. Accessed September 17, 2015. http://www.nybooks.com/articles/archives/1990/dec/20/more-than-100-million-women-are-missing/.

Sen, Amartya, and Jean Drèze. *The Amartya Sen and Jean Drèze Omnibus: Comprising Poverty and Famines, Hunger and Public Action, India: Economic Development and Social Opportunity.* New Delhi: Oxford University Press, 1999.

Sen, Nabaneeta Dev. "Motherhood: Not a Joke!" In *Janani: Mothers, Daughters, Motherhood,* edited by Rinki Bhattacharya, 115–30. New Delhi: SAGE, 2006.

Singh, Bir. "Infant Mortality Rate in India: Still a Long Way to Go." *Indian Journal of Pediatrics* 74, no. 5 (2007): 454.

Singh, Holly Donahue. "Fertility Control: Reproductive Desires, Kin Work, and Women's Status in Contemporary India." *Medical Anthropology Quarterly* 31, no. 1 (2017): 23–39.

———. "Numbering Others: Religious Demography, Identity, and Fertility Management Experiences in Contemporary India." *Social Science & Medicine* 254 (2020). https://doi.org.10.1016/j.socscimed.2019.112534.

———. "Patriarchy, Privilege, and Power: Intimacies and Bargains in Ethnographic Production." *Anthropology and Humanism* 41, no. 1 (2016): 8–27.

———. "Surrogacy and Gendered Contexts of Infertility Management in India." In *International Handbook on Gender and Demographic Processes,* edited by Nancy E. Riley and Jan Brunson, 105–16. Dordrecht, Netherlands: Springer, 2018.

———. "'The World's Back Womb?': Commercial Surrogacy and Infertility Inequalities in India." *American Anthropologist* 116 (2014): 824–28. https://doi.org.10.1111/aman.12146.

Sinha, Bhadra. 2016. "Women Have Right to Be Mothers, Not Surrogates." *Hindustan Times,* February 4, 2016, p. 1.

Sinha, G. S., and R. C. Sinha. "Exploration in Caste Stereotypes." *Social Forces* 46, no. 1 (1967): 42–47.

Sinha, Mrinalini. *Specters of Mother India: The Global Restructuring of an Empire.* Durham, NC: Duke University Press, 2006.

SisterSong. "Reproductive Justice." 2021. Accessed June 9, 2021. https://www.sistersong.net/reproductive-justice.

Snell-Rood, Claire. *No One Will Let Her Live: Women's Struggle for Well-Being in a Delhi Slum.* Berkeley: University of California Press, 2015.

Spiro, Alison M. "Najar or Bhut—Evil Eye or Ghost Affliction: Gujarati Views about Illness Causation." *Anthropology & Medicine* 12, no. 1 (2005): 61–73.

Spivak, Gayatri Chakravorty. "Can the Subaltern Speak?" In *Marxism and the Interpretation of Culture,* edited by Cary Nelson and Lawrence Grossberg, 271–313. Urbana: University of Illinois Press, 1988.

Sreenivas, Mytheli. *Wives, Widows, and Concubines: The Conjugal Family Ideal in Colonial India.* Bloomington: Indiana University Press, 2008.

Srinivas, M. N., and E. A. Ramaswamy. *Culture and Human Fertility in India.* New Delhi: Oxford University Press, 1977.

Strathern, Marilyn. *The Gender of the Gift: Problems with Women and Problems with Society in Melanesia.* Berkeley: University of California Press, 1988.

Street, Alice. "Affective Infrastructure: Hospital Landscapes of Hope and Failure." *Space and Culture* 15, no. 1 (2012): 44–56.

Strong, Pauline Turner. "To Forget Their Tongue, Their Name, and Their Whole Relation: Captivity, Extra-Tribal Adoption, and the Indian Child Welfare Act." In *Relative Values: Reconfiguring Kinship Studies,* edited by Sarah Franklin and Susan McKinnon, 468–93. Durham, NC: Duke University Press, 2001.

Sturman, Rachel. *The Government of Social Life in Colonial India: Liberalism, Religious Law, and Women's Rights.* Cambridge: Cambridge University Press, 2012.

Subramanian, Narendra. *Nation and Family: Personal Law, Cultural Pluralism, and Gendered Citizenship in India.* Palo Alto, CA: Stanford University Press, 2014.

Taylor, Janelle. *The Public Life of the Fetal Sonogram: Technology, Consumption, and the Politics of Reproduction.* Rutgers, NJ: Rutgers University Press, 2008.

Thompson, Charis. "Strategic Naturalizing: Kinship in an Infertility Clinic." In *Relative Values: Reconfiguring Kinship Studies,* edited by Sarah Franklin and Susan McKinnon, 175–202. Durham, NC: Duke University Press, 2001.

Times of India. 2007. Times News Network. Lucknow edition. August 2, 2007, p. 6.

———. 2007. "Adopt a Common Cause: Child Adoption Laws in India Need an Overhaul," November 12, 2007, p. 10.

———. 2010. "Newborn Girl Found Abandoned in Bushes." Accessed April 13, 2022; September 2, 2010. https://timesofindia.indiatimes.com /city/lucknow/newborn-girl-found-abandoned-in-bushes/articleshow /6477256.cms.

———. 2013. "UP to Trigger Explosion: State's Population May Rise to 28 Crore by 2028," June 15, 2013.

———. 2014. "Baby Girl Found Abandoned on Shahnajaf Road." Accessed October 21; August 13, 2015. http://timesofindia.indiatimes.com

/city/lucknow/Baby-girl-found-abandoned-on-Shahnajaf-Road
/articleshow/44892557.cms.

Trawick, Margaret. *Notes on Love in a Tamil Family*. Berkeley: University
of California Press, 1990.

Turner, Edith. "Introduction to the Art of Ethnography." *Anthropology and
Humanism* 32, no. 2 (2007): 108–16.

Turner, James. "A Formal Semantic Analysis of Hindi Kinship Terminology." *Contributions to Indian Sociology* 9, no. 2 (1975): 263–92.

Unisa, Sayeed. "Childlessness in Andhra Pradesh, India: Treatment Seeking and Consequences." *Reproductive Health Matters* 7, no. 13 (1999):
54–64.

Unisa, Sayeed, Sucharita Pujari, and Sujata Ganguly. "Child Adoption Patterns among Childless Couples: Evidence from Rural Andhra Pradesh."
Indian Journal of Social Work 73, no. 1 (2012): 21–44.

United Nations, Department of Economic and Social Affairs, Population
Division. 2019. World Population Prospects 2019: Highlights. ST/ESA/
SER.A/423. Accessed June 3, 2021. https://population.un.org/wpp
/Publications/Files/WPP2019_10KeyFindings.pdf.

United News of India. 2014. "In Landmark Ruling, SC Holds That Muslims
Can Adopt Child." February 20, 2014. Accessed August 13, 2015. http://
search.proquest.com/docview/1500138538?accountid=14667.

United States Central Intelligence Agency. *India*. [Washington, DC:
Central Intelligence Agency, 2001] Map. Accessed May 19, 2022. https://
www.loc.gov/item/2001629019/.

Unnithan, Maya, and Stacy Leigh Pigg. "Sexual and Reproductive Health,
Rights and Justice—Tracking the Relationship." *Culture, Health &
Sexuality* 16, no. 10 (2014): 1181–87.

Vallianatos, Helen. *Poor and Pregnant in New Delhi, India*. Edmonton,
Canada: Qual Institute Press, 2006.

van Balen, Frank, and Marcia Inhorn. "Introduction. Interpreting
Infertility: A View from the Social Sciences." In *Infertility around the
Globe: New Thinking on Childlessness, Gender, and Reproduction*, 3–32.
Berkeley: University of California Press, 2002.

Varshney, Ashutosh. *Ethnic Conflict and Civic Life: Hindus and Muslims in
India*. New Haven, CT: Yale University Press, 2002.

Vatuk, Sylvia. "Gifts and Affines in North India." *Contributions to Indian
Sociology* 9, no. 2 (1975): 155–96.

———. "Purdah Revisited: A Comparison of Hindu and Muslim
Interpretations of the Cultural Meaning of Purdah in South Asia."

In *Separate Worlds: Studies of Purdah in South Asia*, edited by Hanna Papanek and Gail Minault, 54–78. New Delhi: Chanakya, 1982.

―――. "A Rallying Cry for Muslim Personal Law: The Shah Bano Case and Its Aftermath." In *Islam in South Asia in Practice*, edited by Barbara Daly Metcalf, 352–70. Princeton, NJ: Princeton University Press, 2009.

―――. "What Goes On in the Qazi's Office." Lecture presented at South Asia Seminar Series, University of Virginia, September 5, 2003.

Venkatesan, J. 2016. "SC Questions Centre on New Law." *Asian Age*, March 18, 2016, p. 4.

Visaria, Leela. "Deficit of Girls in India: Can It Be Attributed to Female Selective Abortion?" In *Sex-Selective Abortion in India: Gender, Society and New Reproductive Technologies*, edited by Tulsi Patel, 61–79. New Delhi: SAGE, 2007.

Visaria, Leela, Shireen Jejeebhoy, and Tom Merrick. "From Family Planning to Reproductive Health: Challenges Facing India." *International Family Planning Perspectives*, no. 25 (1999) Supplement: S44–S49.

Vlassoff, C. "The Value of Sons in an Indian Village: How Widows See It." *Population Studies* 44 (1990): 5–20.

Volkman, Toby Alice, ed. *Cultures of Transnational Adoption*. Durham, NC: Duke University Press, 2005.

Vora, Kalindi. "Indian Transnational Surrogacy and the Commodification of Vital Energy." *Subjectivity* 28 (2009a): 266–78.

―――. "Indian Transnational Surrogacy and the Disaggregation of Mothering Work." *Anthropology News*, February 2009b, pp. 11–12.

―――. *Life Support: Biocapital and the New History of Outsourced Labor.* Minneapolis: University of Minnesota Press, 2015.

Weigl, Constanze. *Reproductive Health Behavior and Decision-Making of Muslim Women: An Ethnographic Study in a Low-Income Community in Urban North India*. Berlin: Lit, 2010.

Weiner, Annette B. *Inalienable Possessions: The Paradox of Keeping-While-Giving.* Berkeley: University of California Press, 1992.

Widge, Anjali. "Sociocultural Attitudes Towards Infertility and Assisted Reproduction in India." In *Current Practices and Controversies in Assisted Reproduction*, 60–74. Geneva, Switzerland: World Health Organization, 2001.

―――. "Seeking Conception: Experiences of Urban Indian Women with in Vitro Fertilization." *Patient Education and Counseling* 59 (2005): 225–33.

Wilkinson, Steven. "Assessing Muslim Disadvantage." *Economic & Political Weekly* 45, no. 35 (2010): 26–27, 28.

Wilkinson-Weber, Clare. *Embroidering Lives: Women's Work and Skill in the Lucknow Embroidery Industry.* Albany, NY: SUNY Press, 1999.

Williams, Rina Verma. *Postcolonial Politics and Personal Laws: Colonial Legal Legacies and the Indian State.* New Delhi: Oxford University Press, 2006.

Wilson, Kristin J. "Not Trying: Reconceiving the Motherhood Mandate." Diss., Georgia State University, 2009.

———. "Unconceived Territory: Involuntary Childlessness and Infertility among Women in the United States." In *International Handbook on Gender and Demographic Processes,* edited by Nancy E. Riley and Jan Brunson, 95–104. Dordrecht, Netherlands: Springer, 2018.

World Bank Data. 2019. Accessed June 3, 2021. https://data.worldbank.org /indicator/SP.POP.TOTL?locations=IN.

Yngvesson, Barbara. *Belonging in an Adopted World: Race, Identity, and Transnational Adoption.* Chicago: University of Chicago Press, 2010.

INDEX

HOLLY DONAHUE SINGH is Associate Professor of
Instruction in the Judy Genshaft Honors College and
Affiliated Faculty in the Departments of Anthropology
and Women's and Gender Studies at the University of
South Florida.

CPSIA information can be obtained
at www.ICGtesting.com
Printed in the USA
LVHW042110301022
731937LV00005B/68

9 780253 063878